SpringerBriefs in Public Health

SpringerBriefs in Public Health present concise summaries of cutting-edge research and practical applications from across the entire field of public health, with contributions from medicine, bioethics, health economics, public policy, biostatistics, and sociology.

The focus of the series is to highlight current topics in public health of interest to a global audience, including health care policy; social determinants of health; health issues in developing countries; new research methods; chronic and infectious disease epidemics; and innovative health interventions.

Featuring compact volumes of 55 to 125 pages, the series covers a range of content from professional to academic. Possible volumes in the series may consist of timely reports of state-of-the art analytical techniques, reports from the field, snapshots of hot and/or emerging topics, literature reviews, and in-depth case studies. Both solicited and unsolicited manuscripts are considered for publication in this series.

Briefs are published as part of Springer's eBook collection, with millions of users worldwide. In addition, Briefs are available for individual print and electronic purchase.

Briefs are characterized by fast, global electronic dissemination, standard publishing contracts, easy-to-use manuscript preparation and formatting guidelines, and expedited production schedules. We aim for publication 8–12 weeks after acceptance.

Juan José Martí-Noguera

Governing Digital Mental Health

Introducing the 5P Model and the Digital Behavioral Health Expert

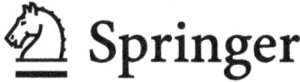 Springer

Juan José Martí-Noguera ⓘ
Digital Mental Health Consortium
Sóller, Spain

ISSN 2192-3698   ISSN 2192-3701 (electronic)
SpringerBriefs in Public Health
ISBN 978-3-031-94762-9   ISBN 978-3-031-94763-6 (eBook)
https://doi.org/10.1007/978-3-031-94763-6

© The Editor(s) (if applicable) and The Author(s), under exclusive license to Springer Nature Switzerland AG 2025

This work is subject to copyright. All rights are solely and exclusively licensed by the Publisher, whether the whole or part of the material is concerned, specifically the rights of translation, reprinting, reuse of illustrations, recitation, broadcasting, reproduction on microfilms or in any other physical way, and transmission or information storage and retrieval, electronic adaptation, computer software, or by similar or dissimilar methodology now known or hereafter developed.
The use of general descriptive names, registered names, trademarks, service marks, etc. in this publication does not imply, even in the absence of a specific statement, that such names are exempt from the relevant protective laws and regulations and therefore free for general use.
The publisher, the authors and the editors are safe to assume that the advice and information in this book are believed to be true and accurate at the date of publication. Neither the publisher nor the authors or the editors give a warranty, expressed or implied, with respect to the material contained herein or for any errors or omissions that may have been made. The publisher remains neutral with regard to jurisdictional claims in published maps and institutional affiliations.

This Springer imprint is published by the registered company Springer Nature Switzerland AG
The registered company address is: Gewerbestrasse 11, 6330 Cham, Switzerland

If disposing of this product, please recycle the paper.

To those who will change how healthcare is provided
Juanjo

Foreword

It is with great pleasure that I applaud the bold vision that Dr Juanjo Martí Noguera lays out in *Governing Digital Mental Health: Introducing the 5P Model and the Digital Behavioral Health Expert*. In this age of rapid digital transformation and growing need for access to mental health care across populations, this work feels especially timely as it addresses the gap between clinical care, digital infrastructure, and policy systems.

The need for equitable, efficient, and digitally enabled mental health ecosystems cannot be understated; I see this work as a pivotal step forward.

By proposing the 5P framework and introducing the Digital Behavioral Health Expert (DBHE), Dr Martí Noguera's work positions governance as a strategic, ethical, and human imperative that harnesses digitally enabled early interventions. Its message that digital mental health must be governed with foresight, compassion, and a commitment to inclusion with the public good always at the forefront is very timely and will resonate with a global audience of policymakers, practitioners, and educators.

It is my view that Dr Martí Noguera's work advances a much-needed conversation that will help shape the next generation of behavioral health leaders.

eMental Health International Collaborative (eMHIC) Anil Thapliyal

Preface: Rethinking Mental Health in the Digital Age

Mental health governance is facing a defining moment. For over a century, systems of care have been shaped by industrial-era institutions, national policies, and profession-bound models of expertise. Today, those systems are being profoundly reshaped by artificial intelligence (AI), digital platforms, and the growing interdependence of global health actors. Yet amid this transformation, a central paradox remains: public health in the digital age is still governed primarily through nation-states, even as mental health technologies—and the needs they aim to serve—move beyond borders.

This paradox creates more than bureaucratic inefficiency. It produces fragmentation, policy inertia, and ethical blind spots. While AI-driven tools, teletherapy platforms, and global apps proliferate, they operate in ecosystems where legal jurisdiction, ethical oversight, and clinical validation are still deeply national. In this gap between digital reach and territorial governance, a new set of risks emerges— among them, platform dependency, unregulated algorithmic care, and the erosion of professional and cultural sovereignty.

The challenge is not simply how to adapt existing systems to new tools. It is how to govern differently. While digital mental health holds the potential to improve outcomes, expand reach, and personalize care, these benefits remain conditional: they depend on ethical alignment, workforce readiness, and governance models capable of navigating complexity across domains—legal, technical, clinical, and cultural.

This book proposes a fundamental shift in how mental health systems are governed: from reactive, fragmented, and institution-bound structures toward a predictive, preventive, personalized, participatory, and precision-aligned framework—the 5P Model. This model redefines "primary care" not as the first point of contact with the system, but as the earliest moment risk can be detected and mitigated. Within this paradigm, mental health governance begins upstream: in data flows, early warning systems, and the coordinated orchestration of support before symptoms escalate into crises.

Crucially, equity in this new landscape is not simply about digital access. The dominant narrative, particularly in relation to low- and middle-income countries

(LMICs), too often equates equity with smartphone penetration or Internet connectivity. But connectivity is not governance. The real risk for LMICs is external governance: when platforms, algorithms, and policy blueprints are imported from outside—developed without contextual grounding, imposed without negotiation, and operated without accountability to local systems. In this model, digital mental health may become yet another vector for epistemic injustice and dependency.

True equity requires governance sovereignty: the capacity of communities and countries to shape the digital mental health ecosystems they inhabit—not just to access them.

To operationalize this shift, we introduce the Digital Behavioral Health Expert (DBHE)—a new professional role designed to bridge clinical, technical, and governance domains. The DBHE is not simply a digital therapist or an IT-savvy clinician. They are a boundary actor, trained to navigate ethical oversight, algorithmic accountability, policy translation, and systems integration. They are a governance catalyst—bringing coherence to a field marked by fragmentation.

But individuals alone cannot fix systems. Governance transformation demands new institutional logics. As the locus of control shifts from ministries of health to app stores, from hospitals to cloud infrastructures, we must ask: Who sets the rules? Who defines safety, trust, and care quality in these new environments? And how do we ensure that innovation is aligned with public purpose—not just commercial imperatives?

The answers will not be found in regulatory checklists or isolated pilot projects. They will emerge through a new governance architecture: one that recognizes care as a shared responsibility across public and private sectors, anticipates risk before harm occurs, and builds capacity for ethical implementation at scale.

This book offers a blueprint for that architecture. It draws on global policy trends, theoretical frameworks, and frontline implementation to propose a model of mental health governance suited to the digital age. It is written not just for clinicians or researchers, but for policymakers, innovators, educators, and system stewards—those who are shaping the next generation of mental health ecosystems.

We are not advocating for a tech-centric future. We are advocating for a human-centered governance of digital transformation—one that elevates trust, transparency, participation, and dignity as design principles. In the coming chapters, we invite you to think not only about what technologies can do, but what systems they require, what futures they create, and what responsibilities they demand.

Welcome to the next chapter in the governance of mental health.

Sóller, Spain   Juan José Martí-Noguera

Acknowledgment

This Springer Brief is part of a research journey that began in 2004, exploring the role of higher education in fostering social responsibility. Mental health care, in particular, demands renewed attention in the digital age—where artificial intelligence is reshaping how care is accessed, delivered, and governed, often more rapidly in discourse than in actual clinical practice.

Since 2018, our efforts have focused on understanding why digital transformation remains marginal in mental health curricula, despite its growing presence in policy and innovation agendas. Thousands of professionals took part in the Iberoamerican Conference on Digital Mental Health, which laid the groundwork for a community of shared learning and exchange. In 2020, many of them contributed to the first Spanish-language *Handbook on Telemental Health* (2022), followed by the *Clinical Casebook* (2022), which captured the contradictions, challenges, and lived realities of digital interventions in mental health care.

Dr. Vanesa Pérez helped direct our attention toward the urgent need for reskilling, while Luis Ernesto Salinas provided a policy-oriented lens that expanded the global perspective. Dialogues with Yolanda Rodríguez challenged us to consider whether a handbook was even necessary—given that digital tools, for all their promise, had yet to become part of everyday clinical routines. Her perspective reminded us not to overstate digital relevance, and to remain anchored in what is actually practiced, not just theorized.

By 2024, digital technologies were still largely absent from most formal training programs. The challenge had evolved: it was no longer just about reskilling, but about upskilling professionals to engage critically, ethically, and strategically with AI—not as passive adopters, but as active shapers of its role in care. *Ethics in Digital Mental Health* (2024) emerged from this context, offering a foundational framework for practitioners navigating the increasingly complex relationship between care and computation.

Dr. Jenny Chávez consistently reminded us to return to what truly matters: care itself. Special thanks are also due to Dr. Claudia Tello de la Torre for her support in the development and preparation of Chap. 2. Her insights and intellectual generosity helped shape and ground key aspects of the discussion. I would also like to thank

Katherine Gibb for her thoughtful feedback during the initial manuscript revision stages—her early observations helped refine the structure and sharpen the clarity of key arguments.

This book belongs to all those who have contributed—not only through their expertise, but through their commitment to values that cannot be automated. It is a collective effort made possible by those who believe care is not an asset, but a human ability that resists standardization.

Language tools such as ChatGPT and Claude supported aspects of the English adaptation of this manuscript. While this book is firmly rooted in the field of digital mental health, it also builds on a longer arc of inquiry. Those familiar with my previous work on social responsibility in higher education and the ethical challenges of digital transformation will recognize a continuity of concerns—and a deepening of critical questions—across two decades.

These pages reflect both continuity and rupture: they extend a line of work committed to interrogating how education systems prepare professionals for a changing world, while responding to the specific disruptions introduced by AI in the governance of care. In this context, what truly matters—human dignity, relational depth, and ethical responsibility—must remain non-negotiable.

Finally, my deepest gratitude goes to my parents and family. Their values—of integrity, humility, and commitment to others—have grounded every step of this work. If this book insists on care as non-negotiable, it is because I have seen it practiced, quietly and consistently, at home.

This work is an invitation to keep the dialogue open. In a time increasingly governed by metrics, protocols, and algorithmic logic, care must not be reduced to data points. It must remain at the center of governance. This book offers not only a framework, but a shared space to reimagine how care can be governed in ways that safeguard what matters most.

Competing Interests The author has no competing interests to declare that are relevant to the content of this manuscript.

Contents

1	**The Historical Evolution of Mental Health: From Nation-State Paradigms to Borderless Care**		1
	1.1	Mental Health Governance: Navigating a Global Digital Transformation	1
		1.1.1 Digital Transformation: A Global Imperative	2
		1.1.2 The Future of Global Mental Health Governance	3
	1.2	Historical Constraints: Geographic Boundaries and Institutional Logics	3
	1.3	Limitations of Traditional Governance Models	5
	1.4	New Governance Players: Tech Companies in Mental Health	7
	1.5	Governance as Power: The Control Question in Digital Ecosystems	12
	1.6	Conclusion: Hybrid Governance and Economic Transformation	13
	References		14
2	**Economic Transformation: Reframing Mental Health Governance Beyond Workforce Metrics**		19
	2.1	Introduction: Mental Health as an Economic Governance Imperative	19
		2.1.1 Economic Evidence for Transformation	20
		2.1.2 Economic Framework for the 5P Model	21
	2.2	Global Digital Mental Health Markets and Economic Transformation	22
		2.2.1 Three Emerging Economic Models	23
		2.2.2 Governance Implications	25
	2.3	Economic Path Forward: Governance Imperatives	25
		2.3.1 From Productivity Tool to Structural Right	26
		2.3.2 Three Economic Domains Requiring Governance Innovation	26
		2.3.3 Governance Approach for Economic Transformation	28

	2.4	Conclusion: Blueprint for Next-Generation Economic Models	29
	References		30
3	**Theoretical Foundation for Digital Behavioral Health Governance**		31
	3.1	Theoretical Evolution of Healthcare Knowledge Distribution	31
		3.1.1 The Clinician-Centered Era: Expertise and Ethical Self-Governance	31
		3.1.2 The System-Centered Era: Standardization and Organizational Control	32
		3.1.3 The Emerging Patient-AI Partnership: Knowledge as Distributed Resource	33
	3.2	Theoretical Framework for Digital Behavioral Health Governance	35
		3.2.1 Platform Ecosystems: Coordinating Without Central Control	35
		3.2.2 Sociotechnical Systems: Aligning Technology with Social Purpose	35
		3.2.3 Learning Health Systems: Embedding Knowledge in Practice	36
	3.3	The Digital Behavioral Health System (DBHS) Framework	37
		3.3.1 Structural Domains of the DBHS Framework	38
		3.3.2 A Layered View: The Platformization Tree	39
		3.3.3 From Architecture to Function: Enter the 5P Model	41
		3.3.4 Why This Matters Now	41
	3.4	Translating Theory into Strategic Priorities	42
	3.5	Conclusion: From Theoretical Foundations to Strategic Governance	43
		3.5.1 Learned Lessons: Where Theory Meets System Transition	43
		3.5.2 Strategic Shifts: From Frameworks to Action	44
	References		45
4	**The 5P Model as a Governance Framework**		47
	4.1	Governance Beyond Technology: The Integration Imperative	47
		4.1.1 Hybridity: Governing at the Intersection of Systems	49
		4.1.2 The Structural Hallucination of Economic Implementability	50
	4.2	The 5P Components as Governance Mechanisms	51
		4.2.1 Predictive Governance: Risk Anticipation Through Data Intelligence	54
		4.2.2 Preventive Governance: Designing Systems that Intervene Before Harm Escalates	55
		4.2.3 Personalized Governance: Contextual Adaptation Versus Standardized Requirements	57
		4.2.4 Participatory Governance: Multi-Stakeholder Engagement Beyond Expert Domination	58

		4.2.5	Precision Governance	59
		4.2.6	From Evidence to Accountability: Diagnosing the Governance Gap	61
	4.3	The Digital Behavioral Health Expert: A Governance Catalyst		64
		4.3.1	Strategic Rationale for the DBHE: Bridging Systems in Transition	66
		4.3.2	Essential Competencies for Cross-Domain Governance	67
		4.3.3	Knowledge Translation Between Regulatory Frameworks and Implementation Contexts	68
		4.3.4	Enabling Governance in Environments of Diminishing Professional Mediation	69
	4.4	Ethical Governance Across Systems: From Fragmented Roles to the DBHE Logic		71
	4.5	Conclusion: Governance as Transformation Catalyst		74
	References			76
5	**Governance and the Role of the Digital Behavioral Health Expert**			**81**
	5.1	Introduction: Bridging Governance and Implementation		81
	5.2	Capacity Building for Sustainable 5P Implementation		85
		5.2.1	Human Infrastructure: The DBHE Role and Core Competencies	86
		5.2.2	Value Governance as a New Implementation Skill	89
		5.2.3	From Ethical Oversight to Cultural Stewardship: Health Ethics in a Digital Age	93
		5.2.4	System Integration: Driving Value in a Fragmented Landscape	97
		5.2.5	Governance Readiness: From Mental Health to Behavioral Ecosystems	102
	5.3	Beyond Implementation: Building a Global Standard for Digital Behavioral Health Governance		107
		5.3.1	Strategic Foundations: Why a Global Standard	109
		5.3.2	Toward a Common Language: The School as First Step	114
		5.3.3	Implementation Pathways: From Concept to Operational Reality	118
		5.3.4	Conclusion: From Capability to Commitment	120
	References			122
Glossary				**125**
Index				**129**

Chapter 1
The Historical Evolution of Mental Health: From Nation-State Paradigms to Borderless Care

1.1 Mental Health Governance: Navigating a Global Digital Transformation

Redefining Mental Health: A Global Perspective
The definition of mental health is fundamentally a cultural construct, deeply embedded in social, economic, and institutional contexts. While the WHO has traditionally provided a global framework, recent research demonstrates the rich diversity of mental health conceptualizations across different regions.

Galderisi et al. (2015) challenge previous narrow definitions, arguing for a more holistic understanding that transcends cultural boundaries. Gerlinger et al. (2013) further illuminate this complexity by examining personal stigma across mental health contexts. This perspective is critically important, as mental health approaches vary significantly across global contexts:

In Saudi Arabia, Almubarak and Alhabeeb (2024) highlight the unique intersection of cultural, religious, and medical frameworks in mental health governance. Khaled (2019) provides additional insights into mental health determinants in Qatar, while Kleintjes et al. (2010) offer a comprehensive view of mental health services across African countries.

Chinese research by Huang et al. (2019) reveals distinct approaches to mental health that prioritize social harmony and collective well-being, with prevalence and intervention models that differ markedly from Western paradigms. In the Arab world, Househ et al. (2019) demonstrate how digital platforms must be culturally adapted, not simply transplanted from Western models.

The dynamic equilibrium model proposed draws strength from these diverse perspectives. As Jiang et al. (2024) illustrate through their work on Chinese mental health text analysis, technology can be a powerful tool for understanding culturally specific mental health expressions.

1.1.1 Digital Transformation: A Global Imperative

The digital revolution in mental health is truly global, not just a Western phenomenon. By 2025, the International Telecommunication Union (2024) projects nearly two-thirds of the world's population will be online, with mobile technology serving as the primary access point across diverse geographical contexts.

Insel (2023) provides critical insights into the evolution of digital mental health care, highlighting key lessons and future trajectories. Naslund et al. (2017) offer crucial insights into digital technology's potential in low- and middle-income countries, challenging the narrative that digital mental health is primarily a high-income solution. Key examples include:

- India's National Tele Mental Health Programme (Government of India, 2023)
- Singapore's comprehensive digital transformation initiative (Singapore MOH, 2023)
- NHS England's (2024) innovative service models
- Innovative AI approaches to suicide risk detection in China (Huang & Hu, 2024)

Systemic Challenges and Workforce Considerations
The global mental health landscape is characterized by significant systemic challenges. Butryn et al. (2017) highlight the critical shortage of mental health providers, a problem that extends far beyond Western contexts. Rathod et al. (2017) emphasize that this challenge is particularly acute in low- and middle-income countries.

Roberts et al. (2018) provide a systematic examination of factors affecting health service utilization, revealing that access is not just about infrastructure but about cultural, social, and economic barriers. Moreno et al. (2020) further illuminate how global crises can expose and exacerbate these systemic challenges.

Reframing Governance: A Multicultural Approach
Traditional governance models have been fundamentally limited by their territorial and institutional constraints. The United Nations Human Rights Council (2020) has increasingly recognized the need for a more inclusive, globally responsive approach to mental health.

Wainberg et al. (2017) underscore the importance of a research-to-practice perspective that respects cultural diversity. This approach emphasizes:

- Predictive approaches that are culturally sensitive
- Preventive strategies that respect local contexts
- Personalized interventions that go beyond one-size-fits-all models

- Participatory mechanisms that include diverse voices
- Precision-based methods that acknowledge cultural variations

1.1.2 The Future of Global Mental Health Governance

The COVID-19 pandemic exposed the limitations of traditional, geographically bounded mental health systems. As Wang et al. (2024) demonstrate through their research on emotional disclosure during quarantine, digital technologies offer unprecedented opportunities for understanding and supporting mental health across cultural boundaries.

By 2025, We Are Social (2025) projects a digital landscape that is truly global, interconnected, and diverse. Our approach recognizes that mental health governance must be:

- Culturally responsive
- Technologically adaptive
- Fundamentally human centered

Conclusion: A Truly Global Framework
This is not about creating a universal model but about building a flexible framework that can be meaningfully adapted across different cultural, social, and economic contexts. By integrating insights from Saudi Arabia to China, from Brazil to India, we create a more comprehensive, nuanced approach to mental health governance.
- Amarante and Torre (2018) exemplify this approach through their work on social psychiatry, demonstrating how local innovations can inform global understanding. The future of mental health lies not in imposing a single paradigm but in creating adaptive, responsive systems that honor the rich diversity of human experience.

1.2 Historical Constraints: Geographic Boundaries and Institutional Logics

Mental health governance systems worldwide developed within two constraining frameworks that continue to shape transformation today: geographic/jurisdictional boundaries and institutional priorities that varied across cultural contexts.

Across diverse societies, mental health services emerged within defined political and geographic boundaries—whether nation-states, colonial territories, or traditional jurisdictions. This territorial organization became the dominant scaffold for care delivery globally, though with distinct manifestations. In East Asian contexts, family-centered care systems operated within community boundaries. In many

African societies, traditional healing practices functioned within cultural jurisdictions. In Western and Soviet systems, state-defined borders shaped service organization. The common denominator was the containment of governance within geographic boundaries, creating enduring patterns in regulatory frameworks and resource allocation.

Simultaneously, mental health governance reflected the institutional priorities of different societies. While Western systems emphasized industrial productivity, other contexts prioritized different institutional values. In Japan, social harmony and group cohesion shaped mental health approaches. In many Islamic societies, spiritual well-being and community integration guided care systems. In China, collective productivity and social order informed mental health governance.

Despite these variations, several structural patterns emerged across diverse systems:

- **Institutional Priorities**: Recovery defined by return to socially productive roles, though "productivity" varied culturally
- **Standardization**: Uniform protocols reflecting dominant cultural and institutional values
- **Professional Authority**: Expertise concentrated in recognized healers, whether Western-trained clinicians, traditional practitioners, or religious authorities
- **Geographic Boundaries**: Systems contained within defined territories with limited cross-border coordination

The post-WWII period saw significant evolution globally. International frameworks emerged through WHO and UN initiatives, while regional approaches developed distinct characteristics. Table 1.1 summarizes the distinct regional approaches to mental health governance that emerged in this period and identifies their primary structural limitations, illustrating how diverse cultural contexts produced governance models with common constraints.

Table 1.1 Regional mental health governance approaches and limitations

Region	Governance approach	Key limitation
East Asia	State coordinated, family integrated	Limited professional resources
MENA	Hybrid religious-medical frameworks	Fragmentation between traditional and modern systems
Latin America	Community based, decentralized	Sustainability and coverage gaps
Sub-Saharan Africa	Task shifting, traditional integration	Infrastructure limitations
South Asia	Mixed public-private models	Urban-rural disparities
Western systems	Insurance and welfare-state frameworks	Institutionalization-community transition challenges

Note: Regional governance approaches reflect historical cultural priorities and geographic contexts, resulting in persistent structural limitations relevant to contemporary governance challenges

As this comparative analysis reveals, despite significant cultural and institutional variations, mental health governance systems across regions have consistently struggled with similar fundamental limitations—particularly their reliance on geographically bounded models and standardized approaches that are increasingly misaligned with the borderless, personalized nature of digital behavioral health ecosystems.

While these approaches reflected diverse cultural contexts, they shared fundamental limitations: geographic boundedness, standardization prioritized over individual context, concentrated authority, and limited adaptivity to emerging needs.

Even international guidance remained embedded within territorial assumptions—presuming services would be delivered and regulated within bounded geographies according to local jurisdictional authority. Such frameworks have proven increasingly misaligned with today's borderless digital environments, where care transcends traditional boundaries and authority structures.

1.3 Limitations of Traditional Governance Models

By the early twenty-first century, conventional governance frameworks—whether centralized state systems, federated models, or hybrid public-private arrangements—proved increasingly misaligned with emerging realities. Systems designed for geographically defined populations struggled to address four fundamental challenges:

Cross-Border Complexity
Traditional governance models face significant structural constraints in a globalized world:

- **Jurisdictional limitations**: Frameworks struggle to address needs that transcend borders—refugee populations, pandemic responses, and digital services that operate across multiple countries.
- **Regulatory fragmentation**: Inconsistent policies across jurisdictions hinder research collaboration, professional mobility, and harmonized standards.
- **Demographic shifts**: Systems designed for relatively homogeneous populations cannot effectively serve increasingly diverse, mobile societies.

The COVID-19 pandemic exposed these weaknesses globally. Most systems failed to address the surge in mental health needs, revealing severe deficits in workforce capacity and international coordination. Digital tools were rapidly deployed without corresponding governance frameworks, creating policy vacuums rather than systematic responses (WHO, 2024b).

Persistent Inequity
Mental health systems remain deeply unequal—both between and within countries. While high-income nations allocate more resources, disparities persist across geographic, socioeconomic, and cultural lines. In many regions, mental health spending falls below 2% of health budgets, with rural and marginalized populations particularly underserved (Patel et al., 2018).

This inequity is not merely financial but structural. Mental health services rarely integrate effectively with education, social welfare, and justice systems. Individuals with complex needs frequently fall between bureaucratic silos—receiving fragmented care or none at all.

Reactive Rather than Preventive Approaches
Traditional governance frameworks primarily respond to crises after they occur. Most systems lack:

- Effective early detection mechanisms
- Population-level prevention strategies
- Systematic approaches to social determinants of mental health
- Integrated responses across health and social sectors

The economic logic of these systems prioritizes crisis intervention over prevention, despite evidence that preventive approaches yield better outcomes and lower long-term costs. Budget allocations remain tied to volume-based metrics rather than well-being outcomes.

Digital Adaptation Gaps
Current governance models have struggled to adapt to digital transformation. While physical health services increasingly incorporate electronic records, AI-assisted diagnostics, and remote monitoring, mental health governance often remains anchored in paper-based, in-person paradigms (Torous et al., 2022).

Key barriers include:

- Licensing frameworks that restrict cross-border practice—even in virtual environments
- Regulatory uncertainty around AI-driven tools and algorithms
- Privacy frameworks ill-suited to cloud-based data storage and processing
- Ethical guidelines that do not address automated decision-making

Meanwhile, commercial digital mental health tools have proliferated globally, many operating outside effective oversight. This creates risks of algorithmic bias, privacy violations, and overdependence on untested interventions. International organizations have outlined high-level principles for digital health governance but have yet to develop frameworks capable of addressing the complexity of platform-mediated behavioral interventions across diverse cultural contexts.

Moving Forward
These limitations do not suggest abandoning existing governance systems entirely—many contain valuable safeguards and culturally appropriate elements. The challenge is creating new governance architectures that preserve public accountability and cultural contextualization while enabling interoperability and adaptive oversight across borders. The proliferation of digital platforms and global data flows makes this transformation both urgent and increasingly feasible.

1.4 New Governance Players: Tech Companies in Mental Health

As digital ecosystems expand, the boundaries of mental health governance have been fundamentally redrawn. Figure 1.1 illustrates the multilayered ecosystem through which technology companies now exercise governance power, the spectrum of challenges this creates, and potential pathways for addressing these challenges.

Traditional systems rooted in nation-state logic are increasingly eclipsed by multinational technology platforms that operate across borders, often beyond the reach of regulatory institutions. These actors—platforms, cloud service providers, and AI developers—are no longer just enablers; they have become de facto regulators, data sovereigns, and global standard setters. Beyond infrastructure, these corporations are actively constructing the paradigms of care.

> **Governance in digital mental health no longer relies solely on institutional mandates.**
> It is enacted through *ambient pushes*—behavioral nudges, interface designs, and notification systems—that shape user decisions *before* they become consciously aware of them. As platforms increasingly govern through UI psychology rather than regulation, ethical oversight becomes both urgent and structurally difficult. Digital nudges—delivered through reminders, framing, feedback, and defaults—function as behavioral regulators embedded in app design. They influence engagement, adherence, and decision-making with minimal visibility or accountability. As Purohit et al. (2023) warn, most digital nudging systems lack ethical scrutiny, leaving users exposed to opaque behavioral influence in contexts that deeply affect mental well-being.

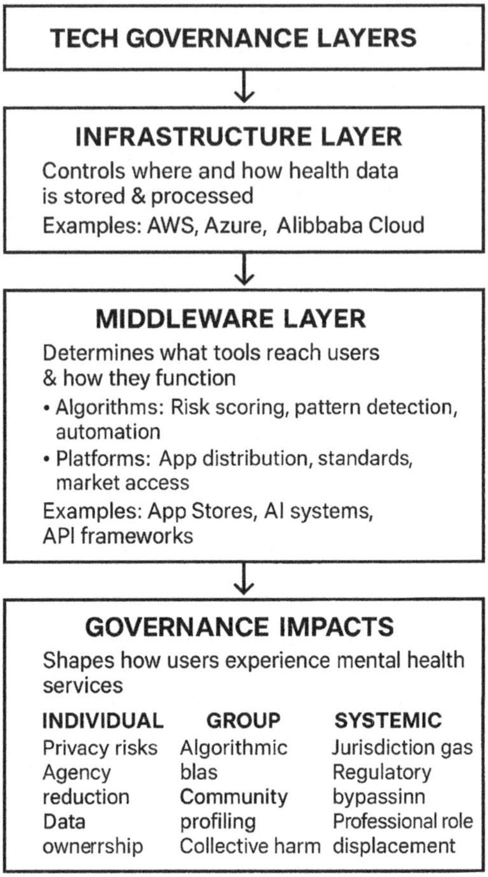

Fig. 1.1 Tech governance layers in mental health. The diagram illustrates the hierarchical governance structure emerging in digital mental health ecosystems. The infrastructure layer controls data storage and processing (cloud providers); the middleware layer determines which tools reach users through algorithms and platforms; the interface layer shapes user experience via behavioral nudges and design patterns. Governance impacts manifest at individual level (privacy, agency), group level (algorithmic bias), and systemic level (jurisdictional gaps, professional role displacement)

TECH GOVERNANCE LAYERS

↓

INFRASTRUCTURE LAYER
Controls where and how health data is stored & processed
Examples: AWS, Azure, Alibbaba Cloud

↓

MIDDLEWARE LAYER
Determines what tools reach users & how they function
- Algorithms: Risk scoring, pattern detection, automation
- Platforms: App distribution, standards, market access
Examples: App Stores, AI systems, API frameworks

↓

GOVERNANCE IMPACTS
Shapes how users experience mental health services

INDIVIDUAL	GROUP	SYSTEMIC
Privacy risks	Algorithmic bias	Jurisdiction gas
Agency reduction	Community profiling	Regulatory bypassinn
Data ownerrship	Collective harm	Professional role displacement

This shift represents not just a change in infrastructure but a transformation in the logics of control and provision. Governance is no longer administered exclusively through ministries of health or public institutions—it is embedded in app stores, code repositories, and proprietary algorithms. While techno-optimistic narratives celebrate the scalability and personalization offered by AI (Olawade et al., 2024), others raise critical concerns. Babu and Joseph (2024), for example, warn that reducing care to algorithmic responses may threaten the therapeutic relationship at the core of mental health interventions.

This tension reflects deeper questions of governance: who defines what care should be in a digitally mediated system—engineers optimizing outcomes or clinicians safeguarding presence?

Companies like Apple, Google, and Meta act as gatekeepers of digital mental health access through app store policies and recommendation algorithms. They determine which mental health tools reach the public, what standards must be met, and which interventions are prioritized based on user engagement rather than clinical efficacy. App stores have become a new form of platform governance, where

1.4 New Governance Players: Tech Companies in Mental Health

inclusion criteria shape the digital care ecosystem without clinical oversight (Hollis et al., 2018). As Lui et al. (2022) demonstrate in their review of physiological monitoring via the Apple Watch, consumer wearables are now embedded in behavioral health data flows—operating at scale and with increasing clinical ambition, despite significant governance gaps.

For instance, BetterHelp, a US-based teletherapy platform operating globally, scaled rapidly during the pandemic by leveraging search engine optimization and algorithmic ad targeting rather than public health integration. In China, WeDoctor and JD Health embedded emotional support services directly into everyday commerce platforms—bypassing clinical systems entirely (Yang et al., 2022; Chen et al., 2024).

Cloud providers such as Amazon Web Services (AWS), Microsoft Azure, and Alibaba Cloud now host the backbone of mental health data infrastructures. They control the physical and virtual locations of patient data, often across multiple jurisdictions with different legal standards. In doing so, they exercise a form of infrastructural sovereignty that reconfigures who holds power over sensitive health data (Luxton et al., 2012; WHO, 2023).

This decentralized storage and processing of mental health data introduces legal and ethical dilemmas around privacy, consent, and jurisdiction. For example, a user in Lebanon accessing a WHO-guided digital depression tool may be interacting with servers in Ireland, algorithms trained in the United States, and terms of use governed by California law—all while falling under no clear health governance framework (WHO, 2024a, 2024b).

These technological shifts have profound implications for data governance. Sadowski et al. (2024) demonstrate, through their analysis of behavioral insurance programs such as *Vitality*, how even nonpersonal, de-identified data can significantly impact both individuals and groups. Their research aligns with the concept of *digital human assets*, showing how fitness tracking and wellness data become valuable commodities—shaping risk assessments and behavioral interventions—while operating largely outside traditional privacy protections. This creates what they term *collective data harms*, where entire groups are affected by governance decisions without meaningful consent or oversight.

This dynamic is especially visible in how private technology companies increasingly act as de facto governance actors within the mental health ecosystem. Table 1.2 outlines the types of tech companies involved, the new governance functions they perform, and the implications these roles have for care delivery and ethical oversight.

The governance roles illustrated in Table 1.2 reveal how technology companies have evolved from service providers into powerful shapers of mental healthcare delivery. This transformation extends beyond traditional regulatory frameworks, creating new challenges for ensuring accountability, transparency, and ethical oversight.

The narrative often presented by these new actors is one of user empowerment—giving individuals direct access to tools, tracking, and support without needing to wait for overwhelmed health systems. In practice, however, this empowerment is mediated by behavioral design strategies, user interface psychology, and opaque personalization algorithms.

Table 1.2 Tech companies as governance actors in mental health

Tech actor type	New governance function	Key implications
Platform companies	Market access regulation	Control which tools reach users and set validation standards
Cloud providers	Cross-jurisdictional data control	Determine where sensitive data resides and how it is protected
Algorithm developers	Behavioral prediction and risk scoring	Create collective impacts through seemingly neutral analytics
Wearable manufacturers	Continuous behavioral monitoring	Transform daily activities into quantifiable health metrics
Social media companies	Crisis detection and intervention	Deploy automated responses or referral prompts in mental health crises, often without established clinical protocols or transparent ethical review

While such systems claim to bridge equity gaps, there remains a lack of structured guidance on how digital health technologies can systematically promote health equity. A recent scoping review protocol aims to identify the existing frameworks and guidelines in this area, noting that without intentional design, implementation, and evaluation criteria, DHTs risk reproducing the same inequities they aim to resolve (Bitomsky et al., 2023).

While patients are "activated" through mobile apps and chatbots, clinicians are increasingly sidelined. Most mental health professionals have not been trained to understand how digital tools work, how algorithms influence care trajectories, or how patient data is used for commercial optimization. The proliferation of dashboards, interfaces, and uncoordinated platforms often leads to cognitive overload rather than integration (Torous et al., 2020).

This results in a paradox: patients are nudged into interacting with data-driven care systems they do not control, while clinicians remain disempowered—relying on opaque technologies they neither selected nor understand. The promise of empowerment becomes, in many cases, a shift of agency toward the system itself.

In contrast, some digital-first care models offer alternative governance pathways by embedding technology within accountable health systems. The Precision Behavioral Health (PBH) model in the United States, for example, integrates evidence-based digital mental health interventions into primary care through structured triage, clinician oversight, and a digital care navigator. This approach demonstrates high patient activation and clinical improvement rates, showing how digital tools can be harnessed ethically and effectively within a governance-aligned framework (Nordberg et al., 2024). These structured models align with emerging US-based recommendations for embedding equity across the entire product life cycle of digital mental health interventions—from inclusive design and real-world validation to equitable commercialization strategies and deployment partnerships (Robinson et al., 2024).

What is notably absent in this transformation is a professional figure capable of navigating these tensions. The Digital Behavioral Health Expert (DBHE) emerges

1.4 New Governance Players: Tech Companies in Mental Health

as a needed profile—trained to understand clinical, technological, and governance dimensions simultaneously. The DBHE can translate regulatory needs into implementation protocols, monitor algorithmic bias in real time, and facilitate ethical data practices in hybrid care environments.

Without this intermediary role, platforms continue to operate without sufficient ethical counterweights, and clinicians are left unequipped to challenge or shape the systems in which they practice. Current models of medical training do not prepare professionals to interrogate algorithmic design, assess platform accountability, or lead governance innovation (WHO, 2023).

The integration of health into the core strategies of global technology corporations marks a profound shift in mental health governance. Companies such as Microsoft, Apple, Google, and Amazon no longer limit themselves to providing technological infrastructure—they are actively shaping the future of care through AI-powered tools, wearable devices, and proprietary health platforms.

These corporations exert influence through multiple mechanisms:

- Platform Governance: App marketplaces like Apple's App Store and Google Play act as de facto regulators, deciding which mental health apps reach users through opaque review policies and algorithmic visibility.
- Data Infrastructure: Cloud platforms like AWS, Azure, and Google Cloud host most digital health services—positioning these companies as gatekeepers of data sovereignty.
- AI Development: Tech giants are driving advancements in sentiment analysis, diagnostic support, and predictive analytics, often setting technical standards that public systems are forced to follow (Microsoft Research, 2024).
- Research Funding: Corporate research agendas increasingly shape academic priorities, pushing research toward commercially viable outputs rather than unmet public health needs (Nosthoff et al., 2021).

This corporate influence creates a deep tension with the governance logic of the nation-state. While governments are bound by democratic accountability and territorial limits, tech corporations are borderless entities whose primary responsibility is to shareholders, not citizens. As a result, decisions about privacy, data use, and algorithmic design that shape mental healthcare are often made in corporate boardrooms—not public health ministries.

For the 5P Model to succeed within this context, governance frameworks must engage—not exclude—corporate actors. These companies are not just stakeholders; they are architects of the current infrastructure. Ignoring their power risks irrelevance. Integrating them into ethical, participatory frameworks is essential to realign innovation with public health priorities.

Future governance frameworks for the 5P Model must:

- Incorporate Corporate Tools: Recognize and strategically integrate platform mechanisms into public regulation
- Establish Public Oversight: Build democratic guardrails around corporate governance systems through transparent accountability structures

- Promote Interoperability: Prevent care fragmentation by ensuring digital ecosystems can work across corporate boundaries
- Address Global Equity: Ensure digital innovation serves underserved populations and does not reinforce existing disparities

1.5 Governance as Power: The Control Question in Digital Ecosystems

The governance transformation described in Sect. 1.4 represents not merely a technical evolution but a fundamental realignment of control in mental health systems. As digital platforms assume governance functions across infrastructure, data, algorithm, platform, and interface layers, the central question becomes: *who designs, controls, and benefits from these new governance architectures?*

Traditional governance frameworks—including many national digital health initiatives—remain anchored in outdated assumptions about jurisdictional control and professional authority. The proliferation of programs like Germany's DiGA, India's Tele-MANAS, and China's WeDoctor signals recognition that mental health delivery must scale, but these initiatives often digitize analog structures without addressing the deeper power shifts occurring beneath them.

What connects these transitional programs is not their technical sophistication but their governance limitations. They expand access without shifting architecture. They digitize services without reconfiguring control structures. They improve reach while reproducing institutional dependencies—from clinical gatekeeping to siloed data ownership. In doing so, they risk cementing rather than transforming existing power asymmetries in mental health (Table 1.3).

This power perspective reveals why simply building digital tools within existing governance frameworks is insufficient. The European Health Data Space and other emerging regulatory initiatives represent important attempts by states to reassert control within platform economies. However, as Staunton et al. (2024) observe, these frameworks often widen "the power asymmetry between the data subject and those deciding on their data access... to the point that the individual has no power."

The 5P Model addresses these power imbalances by redistributing governance authority across multiple dimensions:

Table 1.3 Power dimensions in transitional governance models

Dimension	What appears to change	What often remains unchanged
Access	Digital expansion of services	Professional gatekeeping authority
Data	Digitization of health records	Institutional data ownership and control
Knowledge	Algorithmic decision support	Expert-centered knowledge validation
Infrastructure	Platform-based delivery	Corporate control of technical architecture
Value creation	New digital health markets	Profit-driven resource allocation

- **Predictive governance** shifts control over risk identification from crisis response to continuous monitoring.
- **Preventive approaches** move intervention authority upstream, changing who decides when care begins.
- **Personalized systems** reconfigure decision-making to accommodate cultural and contextual diversity.
- **Participatory mechanisms** fundamentally redistribute who has a voice in governance decisions.
- **Precision-based methods** transform how interventions are matched to needs, challenging standardized authority.

However, implementing this model requires confronting not only technical barriers but economic structures that maintain existing power relations. As we will explore in Chap. 2, the industrial-era economic frameworks that prioritize workforce productivity over holistic well-being continue to constrain innovation and limit access to care.

The future of mental health governance lies not in choosing between corporate and governmental approaches but in developing hybrid models that redistribute control among all stakeholders. This requires economic transformation alongside governance innovation—a fundamental restructuring that values mental health as an intrinsic good rather than merely an instrument of productivity.

1.6 Conclusion: Hybrid Governance and Economic Transformation

The evolution traced in this chapter—from nation-state paradigms to borderless digital ecosystems—reveals a profound transformation in mental health governance. This shift is not merely technological but represents a fundamental realignment of power, control, and authority across global mental health systems.

While frameworks like WHO's strategic guidance (Modules 1–5) remain essential for articulating equity and rights in mental health policy, they are increasingly outpaced by the systems they aim to reform. In digitally networked environments, governance is no longer territorial—it is infrastructural, algorithmic, and often proprietary. These frameworks must therefore be understood not as comprehensive roadmaps but as foundational ethics requiring extension into hybrid, interoperable governance models (WHO Country Office for India, 2025).

The power analysis in Sect. 1.5 demonstrates why governance transformation cannot succeed through technical innovation alone. The 5P Model offers a framework for redistributing governance authority, but its implementation requires addressing the economic structures that maintain existing power relations. Effective governance frameworks for digital behavioral health must:

- **Incorporate Platform Mechanisms**: Recognize and strategically integrate corporate governance tools within public regulatory frameworks
- **Establish Democratic Oversight**: Build transparent accountability structures that maintain public values within private infrastructures
- **Enable Cross-System Coordination**: Develop interoperability standards that prevent fragmentation while respecting contextual differences
- **Ensure Equitable Value Distribution**: Create mechanisms that distribute benefits across populations, not just among those with existing privilege

However, these governance innovations cannot succeed without confronting the economic models that have shaped mental health systems for generations. The industrial-era frameworks that prioritize workforce productivity over holistic well-being continue to constrain innovation and limit access to care. Even as technologies evolve, economic incentives often reproduce the same distribution of power, resources, and outcomes.

The transition to digital behavioral health systems requires more than new oversight mechanisms—it demands fundamental economic restructuring that values mental health as an intrinsic good rather than merely an instrument of productivity. Without economic transformation, governance innovation risks becoming performative rather than substantive.

Chapter 2 will examine how historical frameworks created specific economic models that both enable and constrain contemporary approaches to behavioral health. By analyzing persistent funding gaps, workforce shortages, and misaligned incentives, we will explore alternative economic frameworks capable of sustaining the 5P Model across diverse global contexts. This economic analysis provides the foundation for Chap. 3's theoretical framework, which expands on the dynamic equilibrium model introduced in this chapter.

Together, these chapters establish a comprehensive approach to mental health governance in the digital age—one that addresses power dynamics, economic structures, and theoretical foundations as interdependent elements of effective transformation. The 5P Model emerges not as a technological solution but as a governance framework capable of navigating the profound shifts reshaping mental health in an increasingly networked world.

References

Almubarak, L. N., & Alhabeeb, A. A. (2024). The mental health system in the Kingdom of Saudi Arabia. *Journal of Biomedical Research and Environmental Sciences, 5*(7), 773–778. https://doi.org/10.37871/jbres1954

Amarante, P., & Torre, E. H. (2018). Back to the city, building a social psychiatry network in Brazil. *World Social Psychiatry, 1*(1), 17–22. https://doi.org/10.4103/WSP.WSP_6_19

Babu, A., & Joseph, A. P. (2024). Artificial intelligence in mental healthcare: Transformative potential vs. the necessity of human interaction. *Frontiers in Psychology, 15*, 1378904. https://doi.org/10.3389/fpsyg.2024.1378904

References

Bitomsky, L., Pfitzer, E. C., Nißen, M., & Kowatsch, T. (2023). Advancing health equity and the role of digital health technologies: A scoping review protocol. *BMJ Open, 13*, e082336. https://doi.org/10.1136/bmjopen-2023-082336

Butryn, T., Bryant, L., Marchionni, C., & Sholevar, F. (2017). The shortage of psychiatrists and other mental health providers: Causes, current state, and potential solutions. *International Journal of Academic Medicine, 3*(1), 5–9.

Chen, X., Wu, D., Yu, Y., & Liu, H. (2024). MentalGLM series: Explainable large language models for mental health analysis on Chinese social media. arXiv:2410.10323.

Galderisi, S., Heinz, A., Kastrup, M., Beezhold, J., & Sartorius, N. (2015). Toward a new definition of mental health. *World Psychiatry, 14*(2), 231–233. https://doi.org/10.1002/wps.20231

Gerlinger, G., Hauser, M., De Hert, M., Lacluyse, K., Wampers, M., & Correll, C. U. (2013). Personal stigma in schizophrenia spectrum disorders: A systematic review of prevalence rates, correlates, impact and interventions. *World Psychiatry, 12*(2), 155–164. https://doi.org/10.1002/wps.20040

Government of India. (2023). *National Tele Mental Health Programme: Annual report 2022–2023*. Ministry of Health and Family Welfare.

Hollis, C., Sampson, S., Simons, L., Davies, E. B., Churchill, R., Betton, V., Butler, D., Chapman, K., Easton, K., Gronlund, T. A., Kabir, T., Rawsthorne, M., Rye, E., & Tomlin, A. (2018). Identifying research priorities for digital technology in mental health care: Results of the James Lind Alliance priority setting partnership. *The Lancet Psychiatry, 7*(1), 41–50. https://doi.org/10.1016/S2215-0366(19)30296-5

Househ, M., Alam, T., Al-Thani, D., Schneider, J., Siddig, M. A., Fernandez-Luque, L., Qaraqe, M., Alfuquha, A., & Saxena, S. (2019). Developing a digital mental health platform for the Arab world: From research to action. In B. Maeder et al. (Eds.), *Health informatics vision: From data via information to knowledge* (pp. 392–395). IOS Press.

Huang, Y., Wang, Y., Wang, H., Liu, Z., Yu, X., Yan, J., Yu, Y., Kou, C., Xu, X., Lu, J., Wang, Z., He, S., Xu, Y., He, Y., Li, T., Guo, W., Tian, H., Xu, G., Xu, X., & Wu, Y. (2019). Prevalence of mental disorders in China: A cross-sectional epidemiological study. *The Lancet Psychiatry, 6*(3), 211–224. https://doi.org/10.1016/S2215-0366(18)30511-X

Huang, Z., & Hu, Q. (2024). Tree hole rescue: An AI approach for suicide risk detection and online suicide intervention. *Health Information Science and Systems, 12*(1), 45. https://doi.org/10.1007/s13755-024-00298-3

Insel, T. (2023). Digital mental health care: Five lessons from act 1 and a preview of acts 2–5. *npj Digital Medicine, 6*, 9. https://doi.org/10.1038/s41746-023-00760-8

International Telecommunication Union. (2024). *Measuring digital development: Facts and figures 2024*. ITU Publications.

Jiang, Y., Wu, H., Liu, Y., Zhao, J., & Chen, Y. (2024). Chinese MentalBERT: Domain-Adaptive Pre-training on Social Media for Chinese Mental Health Text Analysis. arXiv:2402.09151.

Khaled, S. M. (2019). Prevalence and potential determinants of common mental disorders in Qatar: A revisit. *Qatar Medical Journal, 2019*(2), 17. https://doi.org/10.5339/qmj.2019.17

Kleintjes, S., Lund, C., & Flisher, A. J. (2010). MHAPP research Programme consortium. A situational analysis of child and adolescent mental health services in Ghana, Uganda, South Africa and Zambia. *African Journal of Psychiatry, 13*(2), 132–139. https://doi.org/10.4314/ajpsy.v13i2.54360

Lui, G. Y., Loughnane, D., Polley, C., Jayarathna, T., & Breen, P. P. (2022). The apple watch for monitoring mental health-related physiological symptoms: Literature review. *JMIR mental health, 9*(9), e37354. https://doi.org/10.2196/37354

Luxton, D. D., Kayl, R. A., & Mishkind, M. C. (2012). mHealth data security: The need for HIPAA-compliant standardization. *Telemedicine and e-Health, 18*(4), 284–288. https://doi.org/10.1089/tmj.2011.0180

Microsoft Research. (2024). *AI for mental health: Ethical guidelines for implementation*. Microsoft Corporation.

Moreno, C., Wykes, T., Galderisi, S., Nordentoft, M., Crossley, N., Jones, N., Cannon, M., Correll, C. U., Byrne, L., Carr, S., Chen, E. Y. H., Gorwood, P., Johnson, S., Kärkkäinen, H., Krystal, J. H., Lee, J., Lieberman, J., López-Jaramillo, C., Männikkö, M., & Arango, C. (2020). How mental health care should change as a consequence of the COVID-19 pandemic. *The Lancet Psychiatry, 7*(9), 813–824. https://doi.org/10.1016/S2215-0366(20)30307-2

Naslund, J. A., Aschbrenner, K. A., Araya, R., Marsch, L. A., Unützer, J., Patel, V., & Bartels, S. J. (2017). Digital technology for treating and preventing mental disorders in low-income and middle-income countries: A narrative review of the literature. *The Lancet Psychiatry, 4*(6), 486–500. https://doi.org/10.1016/S2215-0366(17)30096-2

NHS England. (2024). NHS talking therapies, for anxiety and depression. *Annual Reports*, 2023–2024. https://digital.nhs.uk/data-and-information/publications/statistical/nhs-talking-therapies-for-anxiety-and-depression-annual-reports/2023-24

Nordberg, S. S., Jaso-Yim, B. A., Sah, P., Schuler, K., Eyllon, M., Pennine, M., Hoyler, G. H., Barnes, J. B., Murillo, L. H., O'Dea, H., Orth, L., Rogers, E., Welch, G., Peloquin, G., & Youn, S. J. (2024). Evaluating the implementation and clinical effectiveness of an innovative digital first care model for behavioral health using the RE-AIM framework: Quantitative evaluation. *Journal of Medical Internet Research, 26*, e54528. https://doi.org/10.2196/54528

Nosthoff, A.-V., Maschewski, F., & Baltner, A. (2021, October 25). Big Tech won't make health care any better. Jacobin. https://jacobin.com/2021/10/big-tech-google-apple-facebook-amazon-health-care-surveillance-capitalismdata

Olawade, D. B., Wada, O. Z., Odetayo, A., David-Olawade, A. C., Asaolu, F., & Eberhardt, J. (2024). Enhancing mental health with artificial intelligence: Current trends and future prospects. *Journal of Medicine, Surgery, and Public Health, 3*, 100099. https://doi.org/10.1016/j.glmedi.2024.100099

Patel, V., Saxena, S., Lund, C., Thornicroft, G., Baingana, F., Bolton, P., Chisholm, D., Collins, P. Y., Cooper, J. L., Eaton, J., Herrman, H., Herzallah, M. M., Huang, Y., Jordans, M. J. D., Kleinman, A., Medina-Mora, M. E., Morgan, E., Niaz, U., Omigbodun, O., & UnÜtzer, J. (2018). The lancet commission on global mental health and sustainable development. *The Lancet, 392*(10157), 1553–1598. https://doi.org/10.1016/S0140-6736(18)31612-X

Purohit, M., Fortuin, M., Moorkens, I., Van Hoof, E., & Van Royen, P. (2023). Nudging to change: The role of digital health technologies in behavioral interventions. *Digital Health, 9*, 1–12. https://doi.org/10.1177/20552076231207626

Rathod, S., Pinninti, N., Irfan, M., Gorczynski, P., Rathod, P., Gega, L., & Naeem, F. (2017). Mental health service provision in low- and middle-income countries. *Health Services Insights, 10*, 1–7. https://doi.org/10.1177/1178632917694350

Roberts, T., Miguel Esponda, G., Krupchanka, D., Shidhaye, R., Patel, V., & Rathod, S. (2018). Factors associated with health service utilisation for common mental disorders: A systematic review. *BMC Psychiatry, 18*(1), 262. https://doi.org/10.1186/s12888-018-1837-1

Robinson, A., Flom, M., Forman-Hoffman, V. L., Histon, T., Levy, M., Darcy, A., Ajayi, T., Mohr, D. C., Wicks, P., Greene, C., & Montgomery, R. M. (2024). Equity in digital mental health interventions in the United States: Where to next? *Journal of Medical Internet Research, 26*, e59939. https://doi.org/10.2196/59939

Sadowski, J., Lewis, K., & Bednarz, Z. (2024). Risk, value, vitality: The moral economy of a global behavioural insurance platform. *Economy and Society, 53*(2), 227–249. https://doi.org/10.1080/03085147.2024.2328992

Staunton, C., Shabani, M., Mascalzoni, D., Mežinska, S., & Slokenberga, S. (2024). Ethical and social reflections on the proposed European health data space. *European Journal of Human Genetics, 32*(5), 498–505. https://doi.org/10.1038/s41431-024-01543-9

Torous, J., Myrick, K. J., Rauseo-Ricupero, N., & Firth, J. (2020). Digital mental health and COVID-19: Using technology today to accelerate the curve on access and quality tomorrow. *JMIR Mental Health, 7*(3), e18848. https://doi.org/10.2196/18848

Torous, J., Bucci, S., Bell, I. H., Kessing, L. V., Faurholt-Jepsen, M., Whelan, P., Carvalho, A. F., Keshavan, M., Linardon, J., & Firth, J. (2022). The growing field of digital psychiatry: Current evidence and the future of apps, social media, chatbots, and virtual reality. *World Psychiatry, 21*(1), 8–25. https://doi.org/10.1002/wps.20883

References

United Nations Human Rights Council. (2020). *Mental health and human rights: Report of the United Nations high commissioner for human rights*. United Nations.

Wainberg, M. L., Scorza, P., Shultz, J. M., Helpman, L., Mootz, J. J., Johnson, K. A., Neria, Y., Bradford, J. E., Oquendo, M. A., & Arbuckle, M. R. (2017). Challenges and opportunities in global mental health: A research-to-practice perspective. *Current Psychiatry Reports, 19*(5), 28. https://doi.org/10.1007/s11920-017-0780-z

Wang, S., Zhang, Y., Zhu, H., Shi, M., Xie, W., & Liu, Y. (2024). Understanding emotional disclosure via diary-keeping in quarantine on social media. arXiv:2401.07230.

We Are Social. (2025). *Digital 2025: Global digital overview*. We Are Social and Hootsuite.

World Health Organization. (2023). *Large multi-modal AI models and their governance in digital mental health*. World Health Organization.

World Health Organization. (2024a). *Psychological interventions implementation manual: Integrating evidence-based psychological interventions into existing services*. WHO. https://www.who.int/publications/i/item/9789240087149

World Health Organization. (2024b). *Human resources for health update: Tables January to July 2024 (EB156/HR/update)*. World Health Organization. Available at: https://apps.who.int/gb/ebwha/pdf_files/EB156/B156_HR_Update-en.pdf

World Health Organization. Country Office for India. (2025). *A global review of value-based care: Theory, practice and lessons learned*. World Health Organization. Country Office for India. https://iris.who.int/handle/10665/380713

Yang, H., Zhang, R., Yang, S., Wu, S., Wei, D., Yin, Y., Wang, Y., & Yuan, S. (2022). Chatbots for mental health support: Exploring the impact of Emohaa on reducing mental distress in China. arXiv:2209.10183.

Chapter 2
Economic Transformation: Reframing Mental Health Governance Beyond Workforce Metrics

2.1 Introduction: Mental Health as an Economic Governance Imperative

Chapter 1 established how mental health governance has evolved beyond traditional territorial boundaries through tech-mediated systems. This chapter examines the parallel economic transformation needed to support these new governance realities. The multilayered tech governance ecosystem (Fig. 1.1) and the shift from nation-state to platform-based models (Table 1.1) create not only governance challenges but fundamentally alter how economic value is created, captured, and distributed in mental health systems.

The Economic Paradox in Global Mental Health
Despite imposing an estimated $1 trillion annual cost in lost productivity worldwide (WHO, 2021), mental health still receives disproportionately low investment—typically less than 2% of national health budgets globally. This chronic underfunding has been widely documented by international bodies, including the Organisation for Economic Co-operation and Development (OECD), which emphasizes that mental ill-health costs exceed 4% of GDP in many countries, driven by reduced employment and productivity (OECD, 2021). This misalignment reflects not merely an evidence gap but a deeper conceptual failure in how mental health is economically valued and governed.

Why does this paradox persist? The economic framework that has historically governed mental health systems can be characterized by three defining features:

This chapter was developed with the valuable support of Dr. Claudia Tello de la Torre in its preparation and conceptual review.

1. Productivity-centered valuation: Mental health has been conceptualized primarily as a workforce optimization tool rather than an essential component of human development.
2. Reactive investment models: Resources flow toward crisis response rather than prevention or early intervention.
3. Professional-mediated service economics: Value is defined by billable professional time rather than outcomes or population health impact.

Galderisi et al. (2017) highlight how even the dominant definitions of mental health reflect this productivity bias, reinforcing assumptions that pathologize normal human responses and narrowly define wellness in terms of economic utility. This productivity-centered framework has produced three significant consequences:

- Fragmented, crisis-driven care models that emphasize acute intervention over continuity
- Substantial economic inefficiencies through delayed intervention and system fragmentation
- Deepening global inequities in mental health access and outcomes

2.1.1 Economic Evidence for Transformation

Emerging evidence demonstrates the economic viability of alternative approaches that align with new governance realities:

- High-income contexts: In the United Kingdom, national policy initiatives anticipate improved access, workforce efficiency, and clinical outcomes through the integration of AI in digital mental healthcare (Gardiner & Mutebi, 2025). While full economic evaluations are still emerging, pilot studies and early use cases suggest potential for system-wide gains.
- Middle-income contexts: Brazil and India show that community-based, digitally enabled models fundamentally alter resource allocation while improving access (Amarante & Torre, 2017; Government of India, 2023).
- Conflict-affected settings: The WHO's Step-by-Step digital intervention in Lebanon achieved comparable outcomes to traditional therapy at approximately one-fifth the cost (Cuijpers et al., 2022).
- Planned economies: In China, private-sector platforms have rapidly scaled digital mental health services, with direct-to-consumer models and super-app integrations reflecting commercial strategies typically seen in Western markets (Sabour et al., 2022; Chen et al., 2025).

These cross-context findings suggest that the economic transformation of mental health transcends traditional political-economic divides.

2.1 Introduction: Mental Health as an Economic Governance Imperative

Digital Technologies as Economic Transformation Catalysts
The emergence of artificial intelligence and digital health technologies is directly challenging traditional economic models in three ways:

1. *Value definition shifts* from professional time to data and outcomes.
2. *Investment structures move* from physical infrastructure to digital platforms.
3. *Economic boundaries dissolve* as digital tools operate across traditional jurisdictions.

AI applications do not fit within conventional cost-per-session metrics, forcing reconsideration of how mental health services are valued and evaluated. This technological shift coincides with growing recognition that mental health is not merely an individual clinical concern but a critical societal infrastructure issue.

Misalignment Between Demand, Workforce, and Digital Readiness
Table 2.1 highlights the fundamental misalignment between mental health needs, professional resources, and technological capabilities across global regions.

This data reveals a critical reality: traditional workforce-centered models cannot scale to meet current demands, particularly in regions with limited professional resources. However, digital connectivity now reaches populations where mental health workforces cannot, creating unprecedented economic opportunities for new delivery models.

2.1.2 Economic Framework for the 5P Model

The remainder of this chapter develops a new economic framework for mental health governance organized around three dimensions:

1. Section 2.2 examines how digital technologies are transforming global mental health markets, creating convergent economic patterns across diverse healthcare systems.

Table 2.1 Mental health system capacity and digital readiness comparison

Region	Mental health demand	Workforce availability	Mobile Internet penetration	Smartphone adoption
EU	High (significant increase post-pandemic)	Moderate to low	90–95%	>85%
USA	Very high (substantial increase in help seeking)	Uneven (urban-rural divide)	96%	>90%
ASEAN	High (especially in urban areas)	Low	80–85%	70–90%
MENA	High (exacerbated by regional instability)	Very low	60–80%	60–85%

2. Section 2.3 establishes the economic imperatives for effective governance, addressing workforce economics, data economics, and transition economics.
3. Section 2.4 proposes a blueprint for next-generation economic models that can support the 5P Model introduced in Chap. 1.

By connecting economic transformation to governance innovation, this chapter establishes the financial frameworks required to move the 5P Model from concept to implementation, providing stakeholders with essential economic considerations for navigating the shift toward sustainable, digitally enabled behavioral health governance.

2.2 Global Digital Mental Health Markets and Economic Transformation

Building upon the economic framework established in Sect. 2.1, this section analyzes how digital technologies are transforming mental health markets globally. This transformation represents not merely technological advancement but a profound restructuring of economic incentives, delivery models, and value propositions that directly impact governance approaches.

Convergent Market Patterns Across Diverse Healthcare Systems
The global digital mental health market has grown dramatically, with projected continued expansion through the mid-2020s. What distinguishes this growth from previous healthcare market evolutions is its remarkably similar pattern across fundamentally different economic systems. Despite varying underlying healthcare structures, digital mental health markets show striking convergence in business models, commercialization approaches, and economic structures (Table 2.2).

This convergence is particularly evident in cross-system comparisons:

- Planned vs. Market Economies: China's digital mental health ecosystem shows remarkable similarities to Western market-driven approaches despite fundamentally different political-economic structures. Studies of China's digital health ecosystem show that, despite centralized oversight, most behavioral health apps are privately operated and commercially positioned—often within multifunctional digital platforms. This structural convergence with Western market models is particularly evident in delivery mechanisms, monetization strategies, and user acquisition methods (Chen et al., 2025; Sabour et al., 2022).
- Diverse Healthcare Systems: Across ASEAN, with healthcare structures ranging from highly privatized to predominantly public, digital mental health markets show consistent commercial structures focused on direct-to-consumer models.
- Traditional Investment Patterns: In the Middle East and North Africa (MENA) region, despite significant investments in some Gulf states, most countries still allocate less than 2% of health budgets to mental health, with private out-of-pocket expenditure driving digital adoption.

2.2 Global Digital Mental Health Markets and Economic Transformation

Table 2.2 Global digital mental health market characteristics

Region	Market size	Growth rate	Dominant models	Governance structure	Key market dynamic
North America	Largest	High	Employer focused, subscription	Predominantly private	Digital benefits replacing traditional employee assistance programs (EAPs)
Europe	Large	Moderate	Insurance integrated, reimbursement based	Mixed public-private	Regional regulatory frameworks creating market silos
China	Rapidly expanding	Very high	Direct to consumer, freemium	State oversight with private operation	Super-app integration driving mass adoption
ASEAN	Growing	High	Telehealth platforms, B2C	Predominantly private	Cross-border service delivery challenging national oversight
MENA	Emerging	High	Subscription, out of pocket	Private with public initiatives	Cultural adaptation determining market success
Africa	Smallest	Moderate	NGO partnerships, hybrid	Mixed public-private	Humanitarian and development funding creating sustainability challenges

This pattern suggests that digital technologies are creating market convergence that transcends traditional economic distinctions between public and private, centralized and decentralized, or high-income and resource-constrained systems.

2.2.1 Three Emerging Economic Models

Digital technologies are restructuring mental health economics through three increasingly overlapping models:

1. Platform-Mediated Care

    – Creates two-sided markets connecting providers and patients
    – Extracts transaction margins while reducing search and matching costs
    – Examples: BetterHelp, Talkspace, and regional equivalents

2. Digital Therapeutic Delivery

    – Provides direct intervention without human providers
    – Creates scalability while challenging traditional payment models
    – Examples: Woebot, Wysa, and evidence-based apps in DiGA catalogs

3. Hybrid Human-AI Systems
   - Uses AI for triage, monitoring, and low-intensity support
   - Reserves human providers for complex clinical decision-making
   - Examples: Quartet Health, Mindstrong, Kaiser Permanente's integrated model

These models share common economic characteristics that fundamentally transform behavioral health delivery:

- Decoupling Service from Location: Breaking geographic constraints that previously defined market boundaries
- Enabling Asynchronous Care: Shifting from time-based billing to continuous engagement models
- Introducing Algorithmic Matching: Replacing clinical referral patterns with data-driven allocation

Cost-Effectiveness Evidence

Compelling evidence has emerged regarding the cost-effectiveness of digital interventions when properly implemented and governed:

- In high-income European settings, digital cognitive behavioral therapy programs cost significantly less than traditional face-to-face therapy while maintaining comparable effectiveness for mild to moderate conditions.
- In crisis-affected contexts, a pragmatic randomized trial of the WHO's Step-by-Step program in Lebanon demonstrated a 95% probability of being cost-saving from a societal perspective (Abi Hana et al., 2024).

These economic advantages derive from four key factors:

1. Decreasing marginal costs as digital interventions scale
2. Reduced physical infrastructure requirements
3. Optimization of specialist time through AI-enabled triage
4. Earlier intervention that prevents costly crises

Despite these potential benefits, current market incentives often prioritize commercial scalability over equitable access or evidence-based approaches. The predominance of subscription and direct-to-consumer models across diverse global markets suggests that economic structures are evolving to maximize revenue rather than optimize population health outcomes.

Regulatory Frameworks Shaping Economic Incentives

Funding models for digital mental health are evolving within increasingly diverse regulatory frameworks that shape economic incentives:

- European Union: The AI Act (2024) establishes rigorous requirements for "human oversight" of high-risk AI systems, creating economic incentives for human-in-the-loop models that increase provider involvement but potentially reduce scalability.

- United States: The FDA's Pre-Certification program takes a more market-driven approach, focusing on organizational excellence as a predictor of product quality, potentially accelerating innovation but with less standardized clinical requirements.
- China: Regulatory approaches combine state oversight of data with relatively limited clinical validation requirements, enabling faster market growth but potentially compromising quality assurance.

These regulatory differences create economic arbitrage opportunities where companies develop products in less regulated markets before seeking approval in more stringent jurisdictions. Such practices highlight the need for governance frameworks that can address economic incentives across borders.

2.2.2 Governance Implications

The transformation of digital mental health markets requires governance frameworks that address three distinct economic challenges:

1. Value Distribution Tensions: Current models distribute economic benefits unevenly across stakeholders, with platforms capturing disproportionate value while providers often experience deteriorating economic conditions.
2. Incentive Alignment Challenges: Commercial incentives for engagement and retention may conflict with clinical best practices and evidence-based care pathways.
3. Public-Private Boundaries: The convergence of market patterns is blurring traditional distinctions between public and private mental health provision, requiring governance that transcends conventional economic categories.

The governance implications outlined above demonstrate that market transformations in digital behavioral health are creating fundamental economic challenges that conventional oversight mechanisms cannot adequately address. These challenges—spanning value distribution, incentive alignment, and blurring public-private boundaries—demand a governance response that directly engages with the economic foundations of mental health systems.

This brings us to the economic path forward and its governance imperatives, which must align with the broader transformation of governance structures identified in Chap. 1.

2.3 Economic Path Forward: Governance Imperatives

The economic requirements for effective governance frameworks directly parallel the governance transformation outlined in Table 1.2 (Chap. 1). Each dimension where tech-mediated governance differs from traditional nation-state models—from authority source to evidence standards—has corresponding economic implications. The transition from deliberative processes to rapid iteration, from professional authority to data analytics, and from peer-reviewed evidence to engagement metrics all require fundamentally different economic structures to support sustainable, equitable mental health systems.

2.3.1 From Productivity Tool to Structural Right

Over the past two decades, mental health has been increasingly framed as an instrument to boost economic performance, enhance labor productivity, and reduce public spending on disability. This framing has led to prioritization models based on return-on-investment (ROI) metrics, promoting scalable, low-cost solutions that are often detached from the structural conditions that sustain distress.

Recent macroeconomic analyses by Abramson et al. (2024) demonstrate that the aggregate cost of untreated mental disorders—in terms of productivity loss, secondary healthcare expenditure, and economic exclusion—far exceeds the mental health budgets of many countries. Concurrently, clinical reports from the British Medical Association (2024) describe a functional collapse of public mental health systems, with the UK's case labeled as "a failed generation," caught between structural workforce shortages and ineffective governance.

These findings converge into a critical warning: continuing to measure mental health as a productivity input rather than a structural right generates both systemic failure and moral risk.

This critique of productivity-centered mental health models is not a rejection of productivity itself but a call for its redefinition. When embedded within a preventive and predictive logic, productivity can be reframed as sustainable functionality—supporting long-term well-being, early intervention, and system efficiency. The 5P governance framework encourages metrics that reflect this broader view: not just outputs or ROI but operational value, trust, adaptability, and equitable access. In this model, productivity becomes less about speed or scale and more about coherence, alignment, and social impact.

2.3.2 Three Economic Domains Requiring Governance Innovation

To support the 5P Model, governance frameworks must address three critical economic domains that are fundamentally changing in the digital era:

1. Workforce Economics in Digital Transformation
Traditional economic models based on time-limited, episodic, and location-dependent professional services are being disrupted by AI-enabled care models that decouple service delivery from direct professional time. This transformation has significant economic implications:

- **Productivity Paradox**: Digital tools promise substantial productivity gains but require significant upfront investment in infrastructure, training, and workflow redesign. Many healthcare organizations struggle to realize economic returns during this transition phase, creating resistance to adoption despite potential long-term benefits.
- **Skill Valuation Shifts:** The economic value of different professional skills is rapidly evolving. Technical competencies in digital tool implementation, data interpretation, and remote care delivery are increasingly valued alongside traditional clinical skills, creating economic pressures for workforce retraining and compensation restructuring.
- **Labor Market Disruption:** Platform-based care models are creating new forms of contingent employment for mental health professionals that may increase flexibility but often reduce compensation security and benefits. This shift risks undermining professional stability necessary for high-quality care if not governed effectively.
- **Training Economics:** The economic models for professional education and training require substantial revision. Current training models that prioritize in-person therapeutic skills over digital literacy, population health management, and team-based care delivery create economic inefficiencies in workforce preparation.

Governance frameworks must address these workforce economics challenges by creating economic incentives that reward quality outcomes rather than time spent, support sustainable professional economics during the transition to hybrid care models, and ensure that productivity gains from digital tools benefit all stakeholders including patients, providers, and the broader healthcare system.

2. Data Economics and Value Creation

Data has emerged as a critical economic asset in digital behavioral health, yet current governance approaches fail to adequately account for its unique economic properties:

- **Non-rivalrous Asset**: Unlike physical assets, data can be used simultaneously by multiple parties without diminishing its value, creating new economic possibilities for shared infrastructure and collaborative care models.
- **Network Effects**: The economic value of behavioral health data increases with scale and integration, creating natural monopoly tendencies that challenge traditional market competition approaches.
- **Externality Challenges:** The economic benefits of data collection and analysis often accrue to different parties than those who bear the costs and risks, creating misaligned incentives that governance frameworks must address.
- **Value Capture Asymmetries**: Current economic structures allow technology providers and platforms to capture disproportionate value from health data relative to the patients and providers who generate it, creating inequitable distribution of economic returns.

Effective governance requires economic frameworks that recognize behavioral health data as a quasi-public good with both private and social value. This includes developing economic models for fair compensation of data contribution, equitable distribution of value created through data aggregation and analysis, and appropriate economic incentives for data quality, interoperability, and responsible use.

3. Transformation Economics for Sustainable Change
Moving beyond current fragmented approaches requires governance models with sustainable economic foundations:

- **Multi-stakeholder Investment Models**: Successful governance transformation requires shared investment across public and private sectors, with costs distributed proportionally to expected benefits. Current models that place disproportionate burden on particular stakeholders create resistance to needed changes.
- **Aligned Payment Reform**: Governance frameworks must evolve alongside payment reform that creates economic incentives for high-value digital care. Insurance and reimbursement models that continue to prioritize time-based professional services over outcome-based digital interventions significantly impede governance transformation.
- **Transition Economics:** The short-term economic costs of governance transformation often exceed immediate benefits, creating resistance from stakeholders operating under short-term financial constraints. Effective governance requires economic mechanisms to support this transition period.
- **Economic Sustainability**: Previous governance initiatives in healthcare have often failed due to unsustainable economic models reliant on time-limited grant funding or unrealistic volunteer contributions. Successful governance requires self-sustaining economic models based on value creation and equitable distribution.

2.3.3 Governance Approach for Economic Transformation

The economic path forward requires governance frameworks that address these three domains simultaneously through:

1. *Integrated funding models* that combine public, private, and philanthropic resources in sustainable ways
2. *Aligned incentives* that reward outcomes and value creation rather than service volume
3. *Equitable value distribution* mechanisms that ensure benefits from digital transformation flow to all stakeholders, including patients
4. *Transition support* that provides economic scaffolding during the evolution from traditional to digital models

These economic foundations are essential for the 5P Model to move from theoretical framework to operational reality. Without addressing the economic dimensions of governance, even the most conceptually sound approaches to digital behavioral health will fail to achieve sustainable impact at scale.

2.4 Conclusion: Blueprint for Next-Generation Economic Models

The economic transformation outlined in this chapter is intrinsically linked to the governance transformation detailed in Chap. 1. Together, they form the foundation upon which the 5P Model builds. The multilayered tech governance ecosystem introduced in Fig. 1.1 and the governance roles outlined in Table 1.1 provide the structural context in which economic transformation must occur. Meanwhile, the contrast between traditional and tech-mediated governance in Table 1.2 highlights why conventional economic approaches to mental health are increasingly misaligned with contemporary realities. Addressing this misalignment is essential for realizing the full potential of the 5P Model.

The transformation of digital behavioral health governance requires not only better rules and standards but fundamentally reimagined economic models. The evidence presented in this chapter demonstrates how historical economic constraints have limited mental healthcare effectiveness, how global digital market dynamics are both disrupting and reinforcing problematic economic patterns, and how new governance approaches must address workforce economics, data economics, and transition economics to succeed.

Effective governance for digital behavioral health requires economic models that:

1. Recognize and reward long-term value creation over short-term productivity metrics
2. Equitably distribute the economic benefits of digital transformation across all stakeholders
3. Create sustainable economic foundations for governance structures themselves
4. Address cross-border economic flows while respecting regional contexts and needs
5. Align economic incentives with patient outcomes rather than service volume

The following chapters will build upon this economic foundation to develop the 5P Model in detail. Chapter 3 will establish the theoretical foundation for digital behavioral health governance, providing the conceptual architecture that underpins the 5P Model. Chapter 4 will then fully develop each component of the model—predictive, preventive, personalized, participatory, and precision based—examining their theoretical dimensions and functional capabilities. Chapter 5 will explore implementation pathways through global case studies that illustrate the model in practice.

By addressing the economic dimensions of governance in this chapter, we have established the financial frameworks necessary to support the 5P Model's implementation. Without economic transformation, even the most conceptually sound governance model cannot be realized at scale. The economic considerations outlined here provide the foundation for moving from reactive, fragmented models to sustainable, digital behavioral healthcare systems.

Acknowledgment I would like to thank Dr. Claudia Tello de la Torre for her collaboration in the preparation and conceptual structuring of this chapter.

References

Abi Hana, R., Abi Ramia, J., Burchert, S., Carswell, K., Cuijpers, P., Heim, E., Knaevelsrud, C., Noun, P., Sijbrandij, M., van Ommeren, M., van't Hof, E., Wijnen, B., Zoghbi, E., El Chammay, R., & Smit, F. (2024). Cost-effectiveness of digital mental health versus usual care during humanitarian crises in Lebanon: Pragmatic randomized trial. *JMIR Ment Health, 11*, e55544. https://doi.org/10.2196/55544

Abramson, B., Boerma, J., & Tsyvinski, A. (2024). Macroeconomics of mental health. *SSRN*. https://doi.org/10.2139/ssrn.4793015

Amarante, P., & Torre, E. H. (2017). Brazilian psychiatric reform: Contributions and challenges. *Ciência & Saúde Coletiva, 22*(10), 3267–3276. https://doi.org/10.1590/1413-812320172210.16782017

British Medical Association (BMA). (2024). *Mental health services failing a generation: A crisis in care*. British Medical Association. Available at: https://www.bma.org.uk/advice-and-support/nhs-delivery-and-workforce/mental-health/mental-health-services-failing-a-generation.

Chen, J., Yuan, L., Li, B., Yan, J., & Ren, L. (2025). Precision mental healthcare: Identifying service preferences through discrete-choice experiments in Chinese megacities. Administration and Policy in Mental Health and Mental Health Services Research. Advance online publication. https://doi.org/10.1007/s10488-025-01444-z

Cuijpers, P., Heim, E., Abi Ramia, J., Burchert, S., Carswell, K., Cornelisz, I., Knaevelsrud, C., Noun, P., van Klaveren, C., van't Hof, E., Zoghbi, E., van Ommeren, M., & El Chammay, R. (2022). Guided digital health intervention for depression in Lebanon: Randomised trial. *Evidence-Based Mental Health, 25*, 34–40. https://doi.org/10.1136/ebmental-2021-300353

European Union. (2024). *Regulation of the European Parliament and of the Council laying down harmonised rules on artificial intelligence (Artificial Intelligence Act) and amending certain Union legislative acts, Article 14: Human Oversight*. European Union.

Galderisi, S., Heinz, A., Kastrup, M., Beezhold, J., & Sartorius, N. (2017). A proposed new definition of mental health. *Psychiatria Polska, 51*(3), 407–411. https://doi.org/10.12740/PP/63811

Gardiner, H., & Mutebi, N. (2025). AI and mental healthcare: Opportunities and delivery considerations. *POSTnote 737*. Parliamentary Office of Science and Technology. https://doi.org/10.58248/PN737.

Government of India. (2023). *National Tele Mental Health Programme: Annual report 2022–2023*. Ministry of Health and Family Welfare.

OECD. (2021). *A new benchmark for mental health systems: Tackling the social and economic costs of mental ill-health*. OECD Publishing.

Sabour, S., Zhang, W., Xiao, X., Zhang, Y., Zheng, Y., Wen, J., Zhao, J., & Huang, M. (2022). Chatbots for mental health support: Exploring the impact of Emohaa on reducing mental distress in China. arXiv. https://arxiv.org/abs/2209.10183

WHO. (2021). *Mental health investment case: The cost of inaction*. World Health Organization.

Chapter 3
Theoretical Foundation for Digital Behavioral Health Governance

3.1 Theoretical Evolution of Healthcare Knowledge Distribution

Digital behavioral health does not emerge in a vacuum—it builds on decades of shifting paradigms in how knowledge is created, validated, and distributed within care systems. Understanding this evolution is essential to designing governance models that can adapt to emerging digital ecosystems.

3.1.1 The Clinician-Centered Era: Expertise and Ethical Self-Governance

In the early paradigms of behavioral health, the clinician stood as the central node of authority, meaning-making, and care. Knowledge was concentrated within a professional class whose expertise had been cultivated through formal training, credentialing, and years of experiential practice. Clinical decision-making relied less on codified protocols and more on tacit knowledge—an intuitive, often ineffable understanding acquired through repeated exposure to complex cases, peer supervision, and the iterative nuance of patient relationships.

This tacit knowledge was not easily transferable. It lived in the heads of seasoned clinicians and was shared informally through mentorship rather than standardized documentation. As Polanyi (1966) and later Nonaka and Takeuchi (1995) theorized, tacit knowledge represents a form of intelligence that cannot be fully captured in written instructions or decision trees. In mental health, in particular, where symptoms are context dependent and meaning is co-constructed, tacit understanding was not just a feature of care—it was its very fabric.

Because of this, information flows were narrow and siloed. Patient records functioned primarily as mnemonic tools for individual clinicians rather than as instruments of systemic learning. There was little standardization, limited interoperability, and no infrastructure for shared knowledge beyond the clinician's immediate sphere.

Governance, in this era, was equally interpersonal. It was grounded in the codes of ethics developed by professional societies, enforced through peer accountability and licensure boards. Clinical judgment was considered sacred—shielded from external audit under the premise that only trained peers could evaluate therapeutic intent and effect. This system fostered deep trust and a strong therapeutic alliance but also entrenched a high degree of *asymmetry between patient and professional*. The clinician knew; the patient followed.

Over time, however, this model revealed its limits. Its scalability was poor—each clinician could serve only a finite number of clients. Variability in care quality was high, with outcomes often tied more to individual clinician strengths than to any standard of care. And as mental health demand outpaced available human resources, the model's dependence on tacit, siloed expertise became a constraint rather than a strength.

The clinician-centered era established the ethical foundations of behavioral health, but it also illuminated the need for broader infrastructures—systems that could distribute knowledge more widely, integrate data across cases, and maintain quality and equity at scale. These needs would shape the system-centered era that followed.

3.1.2 The System-Centered Era: Standardization and Organizational Control

As mental health systems matured and the scale of demand grew, a new paradigm emerged—one that shifted the center of gravity from the individual clinician to the healthcare organization. In this system-centered model, knowledge was no longer held exclusively in the minds of professionals but increasingly *codified, standardized, and managed* at the institutional level.

The logic of this era was clear: what could not be scaled through individual expertise might be scaled through protocols, guidelines, and workflows. *Evidence-based practice* became the rallying cry, transforming clinical wisdom into *formalized care pathways* and manuals. This codification was not just a scientific ambition—it was a managerial one. It sought to reduce variability, ensure accountability, and optimize efficiency across large systems.

Governance mechanisms evolved accordingly. Clinical oversight became less reliant on peer ethics and more anchored in *organizational metrics*: adherence to standardized procedures, documentation compliance, and outcome tracking. Inspired by the quality movements in manufacturing and management science, systems began to import tools like *continuous quality improvement*, drawn from the work of Deming and others, to redesign care as a repeatable, improvable process.

This system logic was embodied in new digital infrastructures, particularly the rise of electronic health records (EHRs). These tools promised not only documentation but organizational memory—a shared repository of knowledge across departments, teams, and time. EHRs became more than passive containers; they were integrated with clinical decision support systems that embedded algorithms, reminders, and flags into the flow of care. Over time, these tools reflected what Nelson and Winter (1982) called "organizational routines"—standardized sequences of action that encoded how the system learned and responded.

Yet while the system-centered model brought consistency, it also introduced new tensions—especially in behavioral health. Standardized protocols often struggled to accommodate *the fluidity and complexity of mental health presentations*. Care pathways designed for physical health conditions with linear trajectories did not map easily onto emotional, relational, or trauma-based conditions.

Moreover, in scaling knowledge upward, the system often moved decision-making further away from the patient-clinician encounter. Clinicians were increasingly bound by workflow constraints and metric-based performance targets, even as they were still expected to deliver empathetic, individualized care. This dissonance created what many practitioners experienced as moral distress—the gap between what they knew a patient needed and what the system permitted them to offer.

Despite these limitations, the system-centered model laid essential groundwork for the next phase of transformation. It introduced *information infrastructures*, measurement logics, and institutional coordination strategies that would later become indispensable in digital transformation. But to evolve further, governance would need to escape the rigidity of fixed pathways and embrace a more fluid, adaptive, and context-sensitive approach—one capable of integrating both human judgment and algorithmic insight.

This evolution sets the stage for a new configuration of knowledge and power: the *patient-AI partnership*, where distributed intelligence redefines not just how decisions are made but who gets to make them.

3.1.3 The Emerging Patient-AI Partnership: Knowledge as Distributed Resource

We are now entering a third paradigm—one that neither re-centers the individual clinician nor doubles down on system control. Instead, it disperses knowledge and decision-making across an *expanded network of actors, tools, and interfaces*. In this emerging model, patients, clinicians, and intelligent systems form *dynamic partnerships*, each contributing distinct forms of expertise and agency to the governance of behavioral health.

At the heart of this shift is the growing influence of *artificial intelligence*, particularly large language models (LLMs) and predictive systems trained on massive datasets. These tools are no longer limited to administrative support; they engage directly in clinical reasoning tasks—from triaging symptoms and simulating therapeutic dialogue to offering tailored care suggestions in real time. As Stade et al. (2024) observe, LLMs can now "flexibly adopt conversational styles representative of different theoretical orientations," mimicking psychotherapeutic interaction patterns without having undergone any formal training, supervision, or licensure. This disrupts the historical association between clinical expertise and credentialed human professionals.

But the shift is not only technical—it is profoundly epistemological. Patients today access clinical-grade information through search engines, wearables, and app-based assessments before ever seeing a provider (Lui et al., 2022). This democratization of knowledge challenges the traditional power asymmetry in the therapeutic relationship. Patients arrive to care encounters already informed—or sometimes misinformed—and clinicians must increasingly curate, translate, or counterbalance this algorithmically mediated knowledge flow.

Moreover, digital systems introduce a new kind of contextual intelligence. By aggregating behavioral signals, social patterns, and physiological markers across time and settings, AI systems can detect risk states or opportunities for intervention that are invisible in episodic clinical encounters. This aligns with theories of situated cognition which argue that knowledge is inseparable from the context in which it is applied. In practice, this means governance decisions must now account not only for the content of knowledge but also for its timing, delivery format, and interpretive framing.

This distributed model of intelligence—combining patient engagement, AI assistance, and clinical oversight—holds transformative potential (Calabrese et al., 2021). But it also raises urgent questions: Who is accountable when an algorithm gets it wrong? How are therapeutic intentions evaluated when they originate from code? What happens to consent, trust, and care when digital systems are the first point of contact?

Answering these questions requires moving beyond older models of governance—whether professional self-regulation or system-level compliance—and toward *hybrid, polycentric structures* that integrate algorithmic mediation, ethical guardrails, and participatory design. It is within this evolving logic of shared intelligence that the Digital Behavioral Health System (DBHS) framework takes shape.

This historical evolution—from clinician-centered authority to system-managed standardization and now toward distributed intelligence shared between patients and AI systems—demonstrates the fundamental transformation in how knowledge is created, validated, and applied in behavioral health. As governance has shifted from professional self-regulation to organizational oversight and now toward complex multi-actor networks, new frameworks are needed that can accommodate this distributed, algorithmically mediated reality while maintaining ethical integrity and human agency. The theoretical frameworks that follow provide the conceptual foundation for such governance.

3.2 Theoretical Framework for Digital Behavioral Health Governance

To build effective digital behavioral health systems, we must rethink governance itself—not just who holds authority but how coordination, trust, and ethical oversight are structured. The DBHS framework is grounded in three complementary theoretical lenses: platform ecosystems, sociotechnical systems, and learning health systems. Together, they offer a foundation for understanding how digital systems can be designed to be adaptive, inclusive, and aligned with public health goals.

3.2.1 Platform Ecosystems: Coordinating Without Central Control

Digital behavioral health systems function not as single entities but as ecosystems—collections of apps, data flows, devices, and human actors interacting across organizational boundaries. Platform ecosystem theory helps us understand how coordination emerges in such environments.

Platforms differ from traditional institutions:

- Enable interaction through *shared protocols*, rather than top-down rules
- Create value by facilitating *network effects*, not by delivering services directly
- Allow *third-party innovation* to grow on top of core infrastructure

These systems act as *meta-organizations* (Gawer, 2014)—hybrid structures that combine market, hierarchy, and community logics. This hybridity makes them well-suited for behavioral health governance, which must bridge the gap between clinical care, social support, and public regulation.

From this lens, digital mental health platforms should not be judged by their technical features alone but by how they structure interaction, distribute control, and shape value creation across a wide ecosystem of participants.

3.2.2 Sociotechnical Systems: Aligning Technology with Social Purpose

Technology never exists in a vacuum. Sociotechnical systems theory reminds us that digital tools and human practices must be designed in tandem, not in isolation. In mental health—where context, culture, and relationships are central—this insight is critical.

Key principles include:

- **Joint optimization**: Success depends on balancing technological efficiency with social adaptability.
- **Boundary spanning**: Systems must link across professions and organizations to prevent fragmentation. Behavioral health patients often navigate 5–7 different systems for care (Pincus, 2020).
- **Values embedding**: Technology design always reflects priorities—consciously or not. Governance must ask: whose values are being encoded?

This theory explains why purely technical solutions (e.g., EHRs or chatbots) often fail: without rethinking roles, workflows, and professional identity, no digital tool can transform care.

3.2.3 Learning Health Systems: Embedding Knowledge in Practice

Where traditional systems separate care delivery from research and evaluation, learning health systems integrate them. In this model, every patient encounter becomes an opportunity to generate knowledge, improve outcomes, and adapt system behavior.

Core concepts include:

- **Feedback loops**: Continuous data generation, analysis, and application in real time.
- **Multilevel learning**: Knowledge evolves at patient, provider, organizational, and system levels simultaneously.
- **Real-world evidence**: Practice-based learning complements controlled trials, essential in behavioral health where clinical complexity defies rigid protocols.
- **Adaptive governance**: Oversight mechanisms evolve alongside the system itself.

This perspective reinforces that governance should not merely regulate what exists but actively shape how systems *learn, evolve, and remain accountable* to their communities.

These three theoretical perspectives—platform ecosystems, sociotechnical systems, and learning health systems—provide complementary lenses for understanding how governance must function in digital behavioral health. Together, they shift our understanding from governance as control to governance as coordination; from technology as tool to technology as social infrastructure; and from knowledge as static to knowledge as continuously evolving. This conceptual foundation prepares us to develop the structural architecture needed for effective digital behavioral health governance in the next section.

Each framework contributes specific governance capabilities aligned with the 5P Model:

- Platform ecosystems explain how coordination can happen across sectors without centralized control, enabling diverse stakeholders to collaborate through shared protocols rather than top-down rules—essential for the participatory dimension of the 5P Model.
- Sociotechnical systems ensure technology aligns with care relationships and human needs by emphasizing that digital tools must be designed alongside human practices, directly supporting the personalized and precision components of governance.
- Learning health systems build the capacity to adapt and improve continuously through structured feedback loops, providing the foundation for predictive and preventive governance approaches that evolve based on real-world evidence.

These three theoretical frameworks provide the conceptual foundation for the DBHS framework. By integrating distributed coordination from platform ecosystems, human-technical alignment from sociotechnical systems, and continuous improvement from learning health systems, we can now describe the structural architecture that enables effective digital behavioral health governance.

The practical application of these theories to governance design creates systems that are adaptable rather than rigid, collaborative rather than hierarchical, and continuously learning rather than static—precisely the characteristics needed for effective digital behavioral health governance in complex, rapidly evolving environments.

These principles now converge in the DBHS framework, which will be introduced in Sect. 3.3.

3.3 The Digital Behavioral Health System (DBHS) Framework

The theoretical transitions described so far—from clinician-centered wisdom to distributed, algorithmically mediated partnerships—highlight the need for a new governance infrastructure. Existing health systems, designed for siloed expertise and episodic care, are structurally misaligned with the demands of digital behavioral health. What is required is not just more technology but a new system logic: one that can coordinate across platforms, protect individual agency, and align innovation with public values.

The *Digital Behavioral Health System (DBHS) framework* responds to this need. It provides a conceptual structure for designing, governing, and sustaining behavioral health ecosystems in the digital era. It is not a software platform nor a blueprint for a specific app—it is the underlying governance architecture that enables ethical, adaptive, and collaborative care across traditionally fragmented domains.

3.3.1 Structural Domains of the DBHS Framework

At its core, the DBHS framework integrates three interdependent governance domains:

1. **Traditional Regulatory Bodies**—Ministries of health, licensing boards, and data protection authorities continue to provide the legal and normative foundations of care. They define minimum standards, enforce privacy rights, and offer democratic accountability but often lack the speed and technical agility to govern emerging tools in real time.
2. **Corporate Governance Systems**—Technology companies, platform operators, and AI developers set de facto rules through design choices, platform policies, and algorithmic architectures. These actors manage data flows, implement technical standards, and often shape care pathways without formal clinical oversight.
3. **Multi-stakeholder Frameworks**—Bridging the previous two are hybrid bodies such as public–private consortia, professional alliances, and community-led oversight models. These entities embody the principles of polycentric governance (Ostrom, 2010), allowing diverse actors to co-regulate based on complementary expertise and shared values.

This multi-stakeholder domain exemplifies Ostrom's (2010) concept of polycentric governance—a system where multiple centers of decision-making operate with some degree of autonomy within an overarching set of rules. In digital behavioral health, polycentric governance enables:

- Contextual adaptation to diverse needs and populations
- Experimentation with different governance approaches
- Rapid response to emerging challenges
- Integration of diverse forms of expertise and authority

Unlike traditional hierarchical governance that struggles with the complexity of digital ecosystems, polycentric structures can adapt to rapid innovation while maintaining accountability across diverse stakeholders.

Specific applications of polycentric governance in digital behavioral health include:

1. *Regional data collaboratives* where public health authorities, private providers, and technology companies jointly establish data standards and privacy protocols while maintaining distinct operational roles and responsibilities
2. *Algorithmic oversight committees* that include clinicians, ethicists, patient representatives, and technologists in shared decision-making about predictive model deployment
3. *Cross-border therapeutic validation frameworks* where regulatory bodies from multiple jurisdictions collaborate with academic researchers and industry to establish evidence standards for digital interventions
4. *Digital health commons* that establish shared resources for data, code, and clinical expertise while enabling diverse applications built upon these foundations

3.3 The Digital Behavioral Health System (DBHS) Framework

These polycentric arrangements acknowledge that no single authority—whether governmental, clinical, or technological—can effectively govern the complexity of digital behavioral health alone. They distribute decision rights and accountability across stakeholders with complementary expertise and authority.

These domains do not operate in isolation. They are interwoven through contracts, application programming interfaces (APIs), funding models, professional norms, and ethical expectations. Their interaction creates a complex but potentially adaptive governance ecosystem—one that can align innovation with accountability, personalization with protection, and data use with public trust.

3.3.2 A Layered View: The Platformization Tree

To visualize this architecture, we adapt Van Dijck's (2021) platformization tree as a metaphor for digital behavioral health ecosystems (Fig. 3.1). In this model:

- The *roots* represent infrastructural providers—cloud services, identity systems, encryption protocols—that anchor the system's stability and jurisdictional reach.
- The *trunk* corresponds to intermediary platforms—those that manage data flow, user identity, and service orchestration (e.g., health record vendors, app stores, payment gateways).

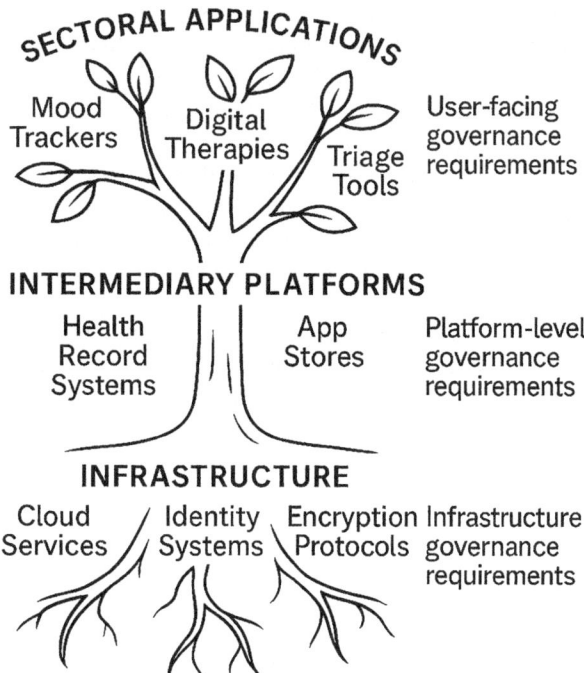

Fig. 3.1 The platformization tree in digital behavioral health showing the layered structure of digital mental health infrastructure, intermediary platforms, and user-facing applications. Adapted from Van Dijck (2021)

- The *branches* are sectoral applications—such as mood tracking apps, digital CBT programs, or predictive triage tools—that interface directly with users and clinicians.

This tree helps clarify a critical point: digital health systems are not monoliths. They are layered, modular, and interdependent. Governance must therefore be attentive not only to top-level applications but also to the invisible infrastructures and platform logics that shape how care is delivered and experienced.

Example

To illustrate how this layered governance architecture functions in practice, consider a typical scenario in digital behavioral health:

A young adult (Elena) living in a rural community with limited mental health resources uses a mood-tracking application on her smartphone. This app represents the "branch" level of our platformization tree—the user-facing application layer. When Elena reports declining mood patterns over several weeks, the app's algorithm (developed by a technology company) identifies potential risk factors and suggests evidence-based interventions while offering a connection to remote clinical support.

This interaction activates multiple governance domains simultaneously:

At the infrastructure "roots" level, cloud services securely store Elena's data according to national privacy regulations while maintaining potential interoperability with her primary healthcare provider's systems.

At the "trunk" level, the app store (an intermediary platform) has enforced basic safety and privacy requirements before allowing the app's distribution, while payment systems enable sustainable service delivery.

At the "branch" level, the app itself implements evidence standards verified through a multi-stakeholder validation framework that includes clinical, technical, and patient representatives.

Without the DBHS framework, these layers might operate in isolation: the infrastructure provider might comply with technical standards but not clinical ones; the intermediary platforms might enforce commercial policies without health-specific safeguards; and the application might follow clinical guidelines without addressing data governance.

Instead, the DBHS framework ensures that polycentric governance spans all layers: regulatory authorities maintain oversight of minimum standards; corporate governance shapes technical implementation; and multi-stakeholder bodies ensure that Elena's experience balances evidence, ethics, accessibility, and personalization—regardless of her geographic location or proximity to traditional care systems.

3.3.3 From Architecture to Function: Enter the 5P Model

The DBHS framework provides the structural base but functionality emerges through the 5P Model: predictive, preventive, personalized, participatory, and precision-based care. These five dimensions, introduced in Chap. 1 and contextualized in Chap. 2, define the capabilities that a digital behavioral health system must deliver to be ethically relevant and clinically effective.

Within the DBHS architecture:

- The *predictive* component leverages data across layers—sensor, platform, user input—to anticipate risk and enable early action.
- The *preventive* function coordinates across stakeholders to intervene upstream, not just react downstream.
- *Personalization* adapts care to individual histories, languages, and cultural identities—not just diagnoses.
- *Participation* ensures users co-shape their care pathways, supported by transparency and relational trust.
- *Precision* demands that interventions are timely, context specific, and minimally disruptive—guided by explainable models, not just black-box optimization.

Together, the DBHS and 5P frameworks form an integrated logic: structure plus function, architecture plus ethics, and infrastructure plus intelligence.

In summary, the 5P Model emerges as the functional crystallization of this theoretical evolution: a model that incorporates the predictivity of data, the preventivity of early interventions, the personalization of context, the participation of multiple stakeholders, and the precision in adapting to specific needs. This functional expression completes the governance architecture, transforming theoretical principles into actionable capabilities.

3.3.4 Why This Matters Now

Many existing digital mental health efforts fail not because of poor technology but because they lack the scaffolding to align innovation with governance. Fragmented apps, disconnected dashboards, and opaque algorithms create a care environment that is cognitively overwhelming for clinicians and often disempowering for patients. Without a unifying logic—without a system—the promise of digital behavioral health remains unfulfilled.

The DBHS framework addresses this gap. It translates high-level principles (such as those found in WHO's Mental Health Action Plans) into operable structures, adaptable across contexts. It allows diverse actors—public and private, clinical and technical, global and local—to coordinate without collapsing into hierarchy or chaos. The DBHS framework offers more than a conceptual overview—it provides the structural logic through which the 5P Model can be implemented in real-world systems. Without this architecture, the five components of the 5P framework remain isolated features. With it, they become interdependent capabilities—functioning together to coordinate ethical, personalized, and scalable care.

In summary, the DBHS framework operationalizes the theoretical principles we have explored into a concrete governance architecture. By integrating traditional regulatory mechanisms, corporate governance systems, and multi-stakeholder participation within a layered structure, it provides the necessary infrastructure for the 5P Model to function effectively. However, before examining each component of this model in detail, we must first understand how this framework transforms the strategic priorities of different governance actors. This next section will explore how stakeholders across the ecosystem must adapt their approach to governance to align with this new paradigm.

3.4 Translating Theory into Strategic Priorities

The DBHS framework has direct implications for how governance is approached across sectors. While its theoretical foundations draw from platform ecosystems, sociotechnical systems, and learning health systems, its real power lies in how these ideas reframe what key actors must do differently.

Three strategic shifts emerge:

1. From Control to Coordination

Governance in digital behavioral health must move beyond jurisdictional silos and professional gatekeeping. Instead, it must enable *cross-sector alignment* among public agencies, private innovators, and community actors. This requires:

- *Policymakers* to support multi-jurisdictional regulatory frameworks that address algorithmic risk, data sovereignty, and value-sharing across sectors
- *Healthcare leaders* to reconfigure organizational boundaries and workflows to support platform-based coordination rather than siloed service delivery
- *Technology developers* to design systems with open interfaces, data interoperability, and mechanisms for shared decision-making—not just user retention

2. From Product to Ecosystem Thinking

Digital mental health cannot be governed through single tools or institutions. Governance must be designed for *ecosystems*—complex environments of apps, data streams, institutions, and users.

This shift implies:

- Designing for interoperability, not isolation
- Evaluating outcomes *across systems*, not just within organizations
- Embedding governance in infrastructure layers—*not just the visible interface*

3. **From Metrics to Meaning**

Traditional governance relies on throughput, compliance, and narrowly defined efficiency. In digital behavioral health, these metrics often miss what matters most: trust, dignity, empowerment, and care quality. The DBHS framework calls for:

- *Governance mechanisms* that balance quantitative outcomes with qualitative insight
- *Algorithm oversight* procedures that center on equity, explainability, and user trust
- *Value frameworks* that reflect the lived experience of patients—not just system optimization

Taken together, these shifts reposition governance as a dynamic, relational process—not a static set of rules or infrastructure layers. The DBHS framework reframes what it means to govern in digital behavioral health: not by controlling every element but by coordinating across systems, aligning values, and sustaining meaning where care is most needed.

Theory alone, however, does not generate change. As we conclude this chapter, we will reflect on the broader implications of these theoretical foundations and strategic shifts, setting the stage for Chap. 4's detailed exploration of the 5P Model components.

3.5 Conclusion: From Theoretical Foundations to Strategic Governance

This chapter has established the theoretical foundation for digital behavioral health governance, tracing the evolution from clinician-centered to system-centered to patient-AI partnership models. Across Chaps. 1–3, a new pattern emerges: the architecture of mental healthcare is already being reshaped by global technological infrastructures, commercial logic, and algorithmic mediation. The question is no longer if digital behavioral health will take hold, but how, by whom, and under what kind of governance.

3.5.1 Learned Lessons: Where Theory Meets System Transition

Lesson 1. The system is becoming borderless—even when governance is not
Technology companies are no longer external actors. They operate cloud infrastructures, control app access, shape user behavior, and increasingly define what is visible, available, and prioritized in mental health services. This transnational ecosystem moves faster than public regulation and is structurally disaligned from

traditional jurisdictional frameworks. Governance, if it is to be effective, must evolve to operate within—not outside—this new architecture.

Lesson 2. The economic model is not broken—it is working as designed

Behavioral health systems have long operated under a model of crisis-response economics. This model tolerates burnout, delayed care, and growing inequity—not as failures but as predictable outcomes of structures that reward volume over prevention, standardization over personalization, and workforce strain over system redesign. The digital transition risks replicating these dynamics unless we design for different outcomes from the start.

Lesson 3. Knowledge is no longer owned—it is negotiated in real time

We are witnessing a shift from clinician-centered authority to algorithm-informed, patient-accessible knowledge ecosystems. LLMs and behavioral prediction tools now mediate care decisions before any clinician is involved. What was once the exclusive domain of credentialed professionals is now part of a fluid interaction between users, systems, and data flows. New professional roles and oversight mechanisms are urgently needed.

Lesson 4. A functional model is emerging—but it needs a spine

Across these chapters, the contours of a new model have begun to appear: predictive rather than reactive, preventive rather than episodic, personalized, participatory, and precision-based. The 5P Model, introduced in Chap. 1 and grounded in the theoretical and economic shifts of Chaps. 2 and 3, offers more than a vision—it provides a structural logic for system-wide transformation. But this model must be implemented through real frameworks, anchored in digital ethics, coordination mechanisms, and new professional competencies.

3.5.2 Strategic Shifts: From Frameworks to Action

To move from vision to practice, digital behavioral health governance must address the three key shifts we identified in Sect. 3.4: from control to coordination, from product to ecosystem thinking, and from metrics to meaning. These shifts are not merely conceptual—they translate into practical governance mechanisms that enable trust, sustainability, and accountability across digital ecosystems.

The 5P governance model presented here does not emerge in a vacuum. It is deeply rooted in the historical lineage of predictive, preventive, personalized, and participatory (P4) medicine, as expanded by Auffray et al. (2010) and further developed by Hood and Friend (2011). Originally anchored in systems biology and cancer care, the P4 paradigm has since influenced a wide range of domains—from occupational medicine to public health and digital ecosystems.

Recent applications of the P4 model in occupational health (Boffetta & Collatuzzo, 2022), telemedicine (Alonso et al., 2019), and systems medicine (Flores et al., 2013) validate its conceptual value and real-world applicability. The 5P Model builds on these foundations and responds directly to the structural challenges and opportunities of digital behavioral health governance.

Thus, the 5P Model is both a culmination and a pivot: it integrates the maturity of P4 thinking while responding to the algorithmic, commercial, and participatory realities of the digital age.

Building on this historical foundation, we must now consider the human capabilities required to implement this governance framework. Even the most well-designed systems require people who can translate principles into practice across diverse contexts.

A digital governance model cannot be implemented using professional profiles shaped for a different era. Successful transformation requires a new generation of competencies, distributed across three key stakeholder groups:

- Digital Literacy for Users and Patients
- Participation in digital care depends on the capacity to understand algorithmic logic, interpret terms of use, and assert agency within systems.
- Digital Leadership for Managers and Public Officials
- Health leaders must navigate complex, hybrid ecosystems, promoting ethical oversight and aligning infrastructure with public interest.
- Digital Clinical Skills for Health Professionals
- Clinicians must copilot care alongside digital systems, integrating AI insights while preserving relational, human-centered practice.

The transformation of mental health systems demands more than upskilling. A fourth profile is emerging—transdisciplinary and system-oriented.

The Digital Behavioral Health Expert (DBHE) is not an operator of technology but a translator of governance across systems. This hybrid role—part strategist, part technologist, and part ethicist—acts as a catalyst for implementing the 5P Model in sustainable and ethically grounded ways.

If the 5P Model offers a compass, Chap. 4 begins to build the map. It defines the principles, actors, and mechanisms that give governance its operational spine in digital behavioral health systems. It explores how ethical alignment, structural accountability, and implementation capacity can be made real—across contexts, technologies, and professional cultures.

The future is not speculative—it is already under construction. The question is how we choose to govern it.

References

Alonso, S. G., de la Torre Díez, I., & Zapiraín, B. G. (2019). Predictive, personalized, preventive and participatory (4P) medicine applied to telemedicine and eHealth in the literature. *Journal of Medical Systems, 43*(5), 140. https://doi.org/10.1007/s10916-019-1279-4

Auffray, C., Charron, D., & Hood, L. (2010). Predictive, preventive, personalized and participatory medicine: Back to the future. *Philosophical Transactions of the Royal Society A, 368*(1925), 2123–2139. https://doi.org/10.1098/rsta.2010.0047

Boffetta, P., & Collatuzzo, G. (2022). Application of P4 (predictive, preventive, personalized, participatory) approach to occupational medicine. *La Medicina del Lavoro, 113*(1), e2022009. https://doi.org/10.23749/mdl.v113i1.12622

Calabrese, M., La Sala, A., Fuller, R. P., & Laudando, A. (2021). Digital platform ecosystems for sustainable innovation: Toward a new meta-organizational model? *Administrative Sciences, 11*(4), 119. https://doi.org/10.3390/admsci11040119

Flores, M., Glusman, G., Brogaard, K., Price, N. D., & Hood, L. (2013). P4 medicine: How systems medicine will transform the healthcare sector and society. *Per Med, 10*(6), 565–576. https://doi.org/10.2217/pme.13.57

Gawer, A. (2014). Bridging differing perspectives on technological platforms: Toward an integrative framework. *Research Policy, 43*(7), 1239–1249. https://doi.org/10.1016/j.respol.2014.03.006

Hood, L., & Friend, S. H. (2011). Predictive, personalized, preventive, participatory (P4) cancer medicine. *Nature Reviews Clinical Oncology, 8*(3), 184–187. https://doi.org/10.1038/nrclinonc.2010.227

Lui, G. Y., Loughnane, D., Polley, C., Jayarathna, T., & Breen, P. P. (2022). The apple watch for monitoring mental health-related physiological symptoms: Literature review. *JMIR Mental Health, 9*(9), e37354. https://doi.org/10.2196/37354

Nelson, R. R., & Winter, S. G. (1982). *An evolutionary theory of economic change*. Harvard University Press.

Nonaka, I., & Takeuchi, H. (1995). *The knowledge-creating company: How Japanese companies create the dynamics of innovation*. Oxford University Press.

Ostrom, E. (2010). Beyond markets and states: Polycentric governance of complex economic systems. *American Economic Review, 100*(3), 641–672. https://doi.org/10.1257/aer.100.3.641

Pincus, H. A. (2020). Care coordination in metal health: Challenges and opportunities. *Health Affairs, 39*(4), 123–135. https://doi.org/10.1377/hlthaff.2019.01622

Polanyi, M. (1966). *The tacit dimension*. University of Chicago Press.

Stade, E. C., Stirman, S. W., Ungar, L. H., et al. (2024). Large language models could change the future of behavioral healthcare: A proposal for responsible development and evaluation. *npj Mental Health Res, 3*, 12. https://doi.org/10.1038/s44184-024-00056-z

Van Dijck, J. (2021). Seeing the forest for the trees: Visualizing platformization and its governance. *New Media & Society, 23*(9), 2801–2819. https://doi.org/10.1177/1461444820940293

Chapter 4
The 5P Model as a Governance Framework

This chapter builds on the ethical imperatives articulated in *Ethics in Digital Mental Health* (Martí Noguera, 2024), a volume developed in response to growing international calls—from WHO, OECD, and national AI strategies—for actionable frameworks to ensure that artificial intelligence and digital systems align with human rights, justice, and social good in healthcare. While that work established foundational ethical principles, this book responds to the next-level challenge: how to translate those principles into scalable governance mechanisms and professional roles. The 5P Model introduced here was conceived as a direct continuation of that effort, moving from ethical reflection to governance design and from conceptual clarity to system-level implementation—anchored by the emergence of the Digital Behavioral Health Expert as a governance catalyst.

4.1 Governance Beyond Technology: The Integration Imperative

What If Innovation Was Not the Bottleneck?
Mental healthcare has been transformed by digital tools—but innovation alone cannot create systems of care. The real challenge is governance: aligning oversight, equity, and safety in a world where demand far outpaces professional capacity.

Mental health conditions affect over 1 billion people globally, while the formal workforce comprises fewer than 300,000 psychiatrists and 600,000 psychologists worldwide (WHO, 2023). This imbalance cannot be addressed by scaling traditional clinical models (Butryn et al., 2017).

As shown in Fig. 1.1 (Chap. 1), today's mental health governance is layered: tech companies exert influence across the infrastructure, algorithm, and user experience layers. The 5P Model is a response to this shift. It offers governance mechanisms tailored to each layer—from data architecture to algorithm oversight and user-centered design. Similarly, Table 1.2 contrasts traditional governance systems with platform-led governance, revealing fundamental divergences in authority, jurisdiction, and logic. The 5P Model helps bridge these worlds.

This workforce gap has catalyzed a deeper transformation: from professionally mediated care to commodified digital services. Platforms now reach millions with minimal clinical involvement. Yet governance has not kept pace. Recent evidence shows that only 32% of clinical trials for mental health apps report adverse events, and 6.7% of users report clinical deterioration—yet most tools lack mechanisms to detect or respond to decline (Linardon et al., 2024). We are deploying systems at scale with limited visibility into risk, impact, or equity.

As behavioral data systems grow more sophisticated, their influence deepens. For example, insurance models increasingly use nonpersonal behavioral data to generate individualized risk scores—affecting people without their knowledge or consent (Bednarz et al., 2024). These systems operate without clinical oversight or public accountability.

The economic logic of care has shifted too. Value is no longer measured in professional time but in user data and engagement. Care has moved from therapeutic relationships to algorithmic flows and from service delivery to platform-based marketplaces.

In high-readiness systems like the UAE, digital infrastructure is in place, yet critical governance gaps persist across domains like equity, clinical oversight, and legal-ethical integration—underscoring that technical capacity alone does not equal readiness (Al Dweik et al., 2024). Meanwhile, AI-based diagnostic tools are rapidly advancing. Meta-analyses show that these systems can now match or outperform clinicians in identifying depression, schizophrenia, and bipolar disorder. Yet few studies assess long-term outcomes, contextual variation, or unintended harms (Rony et al., 2025).

As Adams (2024) demonstrates, the ethical and social risks of digital mental health are often embedded in its complexity itself—emerging not from isolated technologies but from the heterogeneity, interdependence, and distributed control across sociotechnical systems. This perspective reframes governance as a design challenge rather than a compliance task—demanding creativity, negotiation, and systems-level awareness. As Malgaroli et al. (2025) argue, closing the gap between capability and accountability requires a sociocultural-technical governance framework—one that prioritizes inclusion, contextualization, and transparent oversight at scale.

> **AI Performance ≠ Governance Readiness**
> AI is no longer hypothetical in psychiatry. According to a meta-analysis of 150+ models, AI systems now match or outperform clinicians in identifying depression, schizophrenia, and bipolar disorder. Yet governance remains reactive. Most studies overlook how these tools perform across diverse populations or in real-world use. Worse, few report adverse outcomes or clinical reversals. This gap between performance and accountability is precisely what the 5P Model aims to close.

This potential is particularly visible in low-resource settings, where digital mental health tools—when deployed with trained nonspecialists—can dramatically reduce the treatment gap (Faria et al., 2023). Such models exemplify the 5P Model's vision of governance: proactive, scalable, and rooted in inclusion, adaptability, and real-world utility.

The 5P Model offers a way forward. Designed for the shift from workforce-centered to data-centered care, it introduces five interdependent components that reorient governance toward anticipatory, inclusive, and precision-based systems. Each element will be developed in detail in the following section.

This chapter explores each component of the model and the practical implications for system transformation. Framing mental health reform as a governance challenge—not just a technical one—unlocks new possibilities for equitable, effective, and future-ready systems.

4.1.1 Hybridity: Governing at the Intersection of Systems

Digital mental health is not replacing traditional care. It is layering new systems over old ones—technologies, actors, and care logics all interacting in complex ways. Governance must evolve to match.

In this hybrid environment, care delivery blends in-person and digital modalities. Governance spans national regulation and platform policy. Infrastructure links public hospitals to private cloud services. It is no longer a question of old vs. new—*integration is the new imperative*, technically, ethically, and institutionally.

Europe's Trustworthy and Responsible AI Network (TRAIN) initiative exemplifies this shift: policy frameworks like the AI Act and the European Health Data Space are being operationalized through readiness tools—model inventories, bias assessments, and life cycle monitoring (van Genderen et al., 2025). These are not add-ons; they are *governance infrastructure*.

Dimensions of Hybridity in Mental Health Systems

- **Blended Care Models** → Clinical consultations with teletherapy, apps, and AI-based triage

- **Public-Private Collaboration** → DiGA approvals in Germany; WISH chatbot pilots in Qatar
- **Regulatory Pluralism** → National laws and platform policies navigating shared oversight vacuums
- **Cross-Border Data Sharing** → Diverse evidence and privacy norms intersecting across jurisdictions

This hybridity introduces tension: between predictability and flexibility, precision and inclusion. But it also opens the door to *distributed governance*—where responsibility is shared, not centralized.

Rwanda's discontinued partnership with Babylon Health shows the fragility of models lacking long-term coherence. In contrast, Qatar's sustained alignment between WISH, Hamad Medical Corporation, and cultural institutions highlights how trust and ethical integration foster resilience (Househ et al., 2019; WISH, 2024).

As introduced in Chap. 1, hybrid governance emerges when *nation-states no longer govern every layer*. What follows is not disorder but infrastructural coordination. Chap. 5 expands this logic, offering practical mechanisms—*thresholds, role clarity, and feedback loops*—for real-world implementation.

Governance in this context is no longer about top-down control. It is about *enabling integration across domains*: clinical and algorithmic, public and private, and local and global. This is why the 5P Model is not just theoretical—it is structurally aligned with how hybrid ecosystems already function.

4.1.2 The Structural Hallucination of Economic Implementability

"It is not that we lack a workforce. We lack a governance architecture capable of sustaining care at the scale of human need."

For decades, mental health governance has relied on a workforce-centered model that was never designed to scale with population growth. The result is not a temporary shortage—it is the *systemic exhaustion of a model whose economic assumptions are no longer viable*. What is often framed as a "mental health workforce crisis" is better understood as the end of a legacy architecture.

Yet the dominant response has been *digitization without redesign*. This is the structural hallucination of economic implementability: the belief that by digitizing clinician labor or extending reimbursement codes, we can achieve scalability—without transforming how care is governed, structured, or integrated. It is a seductive illusion because it appears rational. But it *merely recycles the logic of scarcity in digital form*.

This hallucination operates in three key ways:

1. It presumes that existing models can be digitized without rethinking governance.
2. It underestimates the hidden costs of fragmented infrastructure, digital exclusion, and misaligned incentives.

3. It assumes that scaling access via platforms equals system readiness—ignoring ethical, clinical, and economic complexity.

At its core, this illusion hides a deeper question: *Who benefits from the collapse of the legacy system—and who absorbs the consequences?* Governments outsource responsibility to markets; markets optimize for engagement, not care; and professionals are asked to bridge gaps without authority or support. The system appears to function but only through increasing precarity.

This creates what behavioral economics might call a *perverse cost-efficiency trap*: short-term savings that produce long-term deterioration. Services are de-professionalized to reduce labor costs. Care is automated without governance capacity. Digital tools proliferate in isolation, untethered from strategy or infrastructure.

If left unchallenged, this illusion will deform the future of digital mental health. We risk reproducing a brittle system—this time in code. The 5P Model rejects this logic. It begins from a different question: *What kind of system would we build if we were not trying to scale the past?*

From Hallucination to Governance: A Model with Evidence

The 5P Model is not merely a critique—it is a structured and evidence-based governance alternative. It offers five components—predictive, preventive, personalized, participatory, and precision-based—that reframe implementability as a matter of *infrastructure, ethics, and participation*. These are not abstract ideals but mechanisms grounded in cases, validated in practice, and designed to govern transformation—not presume it.

In response to these structural failures—the hollowing out of workforce-centered models, the commodification of care, and the governance void around hybrid systems—the 5P Model reorients digital mental health governance toward a new foundation. It is not a technical framework but a governance scaffold that aligns implementation with ethical, clinical, and infrastructural realities. Each component of the model addresses a specific gap exposed in current systems: from predictive oversight and preventive design to participatory mechanisms and precision-based adaptation. What follows is not just a theoretical model but a set of governance mechanisms grounded in real-world cases and implementation logic.

4.2 The 5P Components as Governance Mechanisms

The 5P Model reconceptualizes governance for behavioral health systems increasingly operating beyond traditional professional mediation. Each component functions as a governance mechanism that addresses a core challenge in the shift from workforce-centered to data-centered care: oversight gaps, structural fragmentation, inequity, institutional inertia, and asymmetries in risk distribution.

> As outlined in Chaps. 1 and 3, the 5P Model redefines "primary care" as *anticipatory rather than reactive*—intervening before symptoms escalate. This shift relies on AI-driven detection, digital nudges, and upstream support networks. Traditional clinical care remains vital but moves to second line, activated only when preventive systems are bypassed or exceeded.

Simulation studies by Iorfino et al. (2021) demonstrate that this redefined care model—based on technology-enabled coordination and upstream intervention—significantly outperforms both expanded capacity and standard telehealth in reducing suicidality, emergency presentations, and psychological distress. Their findings underscore that population-level outcomes are not determined by access alone but by the governance architecture surrounding that access.

Ethical considerations are not supplementary but foundational to the 5P Model's logic. As Martí-Noguera (2024) argues, governance in digital mental health must prioritize justice, transparency, and collective well-being across systems that increasingly operate beyond clinical oversight.

While models like value-based care have attempted to reorient healthcare systems around the concept of value, their operationalization often remains vague or narrowly tied to financial incentives. The 5P Model addresses this gap by translating ethical and strategic aspirations into structured governance mechanisms—linking system design to real-world accountability.

Each "P" in the model—*predictive*, preventive, *personalized*, *participatory*, and *precise*—represents not just a care philosophy but a functional governance response to digital complexity. These mechanisms enable systems to move beyond legacy structures and support cross-sector oversight of tools operating at population scale.

These components are not theoretical—they are already being used to reconfigure digital governance across regions such as Singapore, Germany, and Rwanda. Table 4.1 synthesizes this alignment, showing how each component translates into system-level action.

Each component of the 5P Model addresses specific governance challenges created by the tech governance structures outlined in Chap. 1. Where Table 1.1 identified how different tech actors have assumed governance roles in mental health, the 5P Model provides targeted governance mechanisms to ensure these roles serve public interest, clinical effectiveness, and ethical oversight. Similarly, where Table 1.2 highlighted the tensions between traditional and tech-mediated governance

4.2 The 5P Components as Governance Mechanisms

Table 4.1 The 5P Model as a governance framework

5P governance mechanism	Governance purpose	Mechanisms	Core processes	Example implementation
Predictive governance	Anticipate and intervene before risks materialize using data and AI	• Algorithmic pattern detection • Risk modeling systems • Early signal detection protocols	Continuous analysis of digital system data, identifying behavioral anomalies, translating data points into actionable risk indicators	Singapore's AI-powered early detection infrastructure tracking population-level behavioral data
Preventive governance	Intervene early to address potential problems before they escalate	• Tiered intervention protocols • Just-in-time resource allocation • Upstream support networks	Structured intervention approaches, mobilizing appropriate resources, creating coordinated support ecosystems	China's Tree Hole Rescue Team using social media scanning and volunteer response networks
Personalized governance	Adapt oversight to contextual and cultural realities across diverse populations	• Context-sensitive oversight • Risk-calibrated regulation • Culturally adaptive standards	Sociocultural mapping, differential risk assessment, localized standards development	Qatar's World Mental Health Study integrating epidemiological, clinical, and sociocultural data
Participatory governance	Ensure accountability through inclusive, transparent decision-making	• Multi-stakeholder governance bodies • Lived experience integration • Decision transparency	Deliberative engagement, incorporating first-hand insights, creating public visibility into decision-making	Australian Digital Social and Emotional Wellbeing (d-SEWB) initiative: CBPR transformed a top-down digital mental health project into a ground-up, community-guided governance process, leading to the national WellMob platform and reframing national policy toward Indigenous-defined digital wellbeing frameworks (Bennett-Levy et al., 2021)
Precision governance	Calibrate requirements to risk, use case, and impact	• Risk-calibrated frameworks • Evidence-proportionate regulation • Implementation-sensitive standards	Precision risk stratification, population-equitable validation, adaptable oversight	Germany's DiGA model of performance-based regulation for digital health applications

approaches, the 5P Model offers integrative mechanisms that retain democratic accountability while enabling technological innovation.

4.2.1 Predictive Governance: Risk Anticipation Through Data Intelligence

Predictive governance uses data analytics and AI to identify emerging risks before they manifest as clinical problems. In data-rich environments operating at scale, traditional governance—relying on lagging indicators such as adverse events, complaints, or post hoc investigations—cannot protect users in real time. Instead, predictive governance employs continuous monitoring and pattern recognition to detect early warning signs and enable proactive intervention.

This governance logic rests on three core pillars:

- **Algorithmic pattern detection** → Continuous analysis of digital system data across user populations to identify behavioral, usage, or performance anomalies that predict potential problems
- **Risk modeling systems** → Predictive algorithms that translate disparate data points into actionable risk indicators before traditional clinical thresholds would be triggered
- **Early signal detection protocols** → Structured methods for differentiating meaningful signals from noise in complex behavioral data streams

Singapore's national mental health strategy exemplifies this approach. Its AI-powered early detection infrastructure analyzes population-level behavioral data to identify emerging mental health needs before they reach crisis points, triggering alerts and mobilizing responses well before traditional systems would detect a problem (Singapore MOH, 2023).

Wearable devices such as the Apple Watch further illustrate both the promise and pitfalls of predictive governance. Lui et al. (2022) provide systematic evidence that physiological signals—especially heart rate variability (HRV), sleep duration, and energy expenditure—can predict emotional and psychological states. However, Adil et al. (2024) caution that without clinical-grade validation, contextual calibration, and integrated response mechanisms, these prediction systems risk producing false signals, overestimated risks, or unsupervised self-diagnosis. Their findings reinforce the need for governance frameworks that distinguish between data collection and actionable prediction.

Measurement-based care (MBC) provides a further applied case of preventive governance. When embedded into systemic workflows and supported by governance structures—not just left to clinician discretion—MBC can transform real-time symptom monitoring into predictive action. Evidence from youth services and general mental health contexts demonstrates that MBC only achieves this potential when fully integrated into training, reimbursement, and feedback systems—not simply promoted as a clinical tool (Whitmyre et al., 2024; van Sonsbeek et al., 2023).

Ultimately, *predictive governance shifts the timeframe of responsibility*. Rather than determining what went wrong after failure, it identifies what might go wrong before problems manifest—designing systems that continuously analyze patterns to enable upstream action. In digital behavioral health, where millions of interactions unfold beyond clinical view, this forward-looking capability is essential.

While prediction identifies potential problems, a complementary governance approach is needed to act on these insights effectively. This is where *preventive governance* becomes essential, as we will explore in Sect. 4.2.5.

4.2.2 Preventive Governance: Designing Systems that Intervene Before Harm Escalates

Preventive governance focuses on creating intervention systems that address potential problems before they escalate into clinical crises or cause harm. While predictive governance (Sect. 4.2.1) identifies emerging risks through data and pattern analysis, preventive governance establishes the structures, protocols, and interventions that act on these insights effectively.

In the context of digital behavioral health, preventive governance means designing systems that can deliver appropriate supports, nudges, and interventions at the earliest effective moment—often before problems would become visible in traditional care pathways. This approach transforms mental healthcare from crisis response to proactive support.

Preventive governance operates through three essential mechanisms:

- **Tiered intervention protocols** → Structured, evidence-based approaches that match the appropriate level of intervention to identified risk levels, ensuring proportionate responses
- **Just-in-time resource allocation** → Systems that mobilize appropriate clinical, social, and technological resources at the right moment to prevent escalation
- **Upstream support networks** → Coordinated ecosystems of professional and nonprofessional supports that can be activated based on early warning signals

China's Tree Hole Rescue Team offers a compelling example of preventive governance in action. By combining natural language processing for social media scanning with a coordinated volunteer response network, they translate suicide risk detection into timely intervention—preventing crises rather than managing them (Huang & Hu, 2024). Similarly, measurement-based care (MBC), when integrated into system-wide workflows and decision supports, transforms symptom tracking from passive monitoring into active prevention (Whitmyre et al., 2024).

Preventive governance faces distinct implementation challenges. Digital intervention tools such as behavioral nudges, reminders, and wellness prompts can shift user behavior subtly but significantly—raising questions about consent, autonomy, and the ethically appropriate threshold for intervention. Without proper governance, early intervention can easily become surveillance, creating what Ceballos-Espinoza (2024) describe as "digital behavioral residue" that follows users across contexts.

Preventive governance reframes mental health oversight around upstream protection—intervening before distress escalates or becomes clinically visible. In the context of digital behavioral health, this means governing systems that monitor, interpret, and respond to behavioral data in real time—often without direct professional mediation.

Traditional regulatory systems operate on lagging indicators: adverse events, complaints, or diagnostic thresholds. In contrast, digital systems increasingly rely on predictive analytics, passive data collection, and behavioral nudging to infer risk states and trigger interventions early. Governance must evolve to match this new paradigm.

Preventive governance rests on three core mechanisms:

- Algorithmic risk monitoring → Ongoing detection of usage or behavioral anomalies across populations
- Early warning systems → AI models that flag escalation risk before it translates into harm
- Anticipatory intervention protocols → Structured responses built to act upstream of clinical diagnosis or system engagement

Singapore's national mental health strategy offers a compelling model: its population-level monitoring system tracks behavioral patterns and activates alerts before traditional care systems detect deterioration (Singapore MOH, 2023). Similarly, measurement-based care (MBC), when integrated into system-wide workflows, enables proactive adjustment of care plans based on symptom trajectories (Whitmyre et al., 2024).

However, this approach is not without risk. Wearables, for example, offer early physiological indicators (e.g., HRV, sleep disruption), but without clinical validation or interpretability, they may produce false reassurance or anxiety (Adil et al., 2024). Behavioral nudges, widely used in wellness and engagement apps, can shift user behavior subtly—raising ethical questions about consent, manipulation, and autonomy.

> **Important Preventive ≠ Protective Without Governance**
> Digital prevention systems can easily become:
>
> - Monitoring without care → Surveillance tools that collect data without providing support
> - Prediction without context → Risk models that profile users based on opaque signals
> - Nudging without transparency → Behavioral steering mechanisms without user awareness or consent

(continued)

> Preventive governance must:
>
> - Define intervention thresholds for nonclinical systems
> - Regulate data use, model bias, and user recourse
> - Ensure nonprofessional tools have ethical backstops, especially when used at population scale
>
> The logic of prevention must be governed, not outsourced to platforms or delegated to users. Without structured oversight, what appears as early intervention can quickly become structural abandonment disguised as empowerment.

While preventive governance protects systems from collapse, implementing it requires professionals who can operate across clinical, technical, and regulatory boundaries. This is the role of the Digital Behavioral Health Expert, introduced in the next section.

4.2.3 Personalized Governance: Contextual Adaptation Versus Standardized Requirements

Personalized governance creates frameworks that calibrate oversight based on context, risk, and user diversity—rather than applying uniform rules to heterogeneous populations and settings. This addresses a core governance gap in digital behavioral health: the tension between standardization and contextual relevance.

Traditional oversight mechanisms often enforce blanket requirements across all systems, populations, and environments. While designed for consistency, this logic disregards key differences in cultural norms, risk exposure, and infrastructure capacity—creating inefficiencies, blind spots, and unintended harms.

Personalized governance reconfigures this logic by establishing:

- **Context-sensitive oversight** → Adapting governance requirements to population characteristics, cultural frameworks, and implementation conditions
- **Risk-calibrated regulation** → Aligning oversight intensity with the potential harm, complexity, and variability of specific use cases
- **Culturally adaptive standards** → Maintaining core safety expectations while integrating diverse health beliefs and behavioral norms

Qatar's World Mental Health Study exemplifies this approach. By combining epidemiological, clinical, and sociocultural data, it develops governance logic that reflects population realities—not just system assumptions. As Khaled et al. (2024) observe, universal regulatory models fail to detect "hidden" morbidity in communities where stigma or underreporting distorts clinical visibility. The Qatar model avoids this distortion by building oversight around cultural patterns and local epistemologies. This advances the WHO's long-standing critique of governance systems that equate standardization with equity—when, in fact, uncalibrated governance often amplifies exclusion.

This is not merely about customizing care or translating tools. In digital behavioral health, *personalization becomes a governance responsibility*. Platforms and algorithms now shape mental health journeys across legal, linguistic, and social contexts. Without frameworks tailored to these variations, oversight becomes either *too rigid to support innovation* or *too generic to ensure protection*.

Governance Insight

Personalization is not about clinical customization alone—it is about recalibrating governance standards to reflect the lived diversity of systems and populations.

But contextual adaptation is not enough. Governance must also be *structurally accountable* to the communities it serves. That requires participatory design—governance with people, not just for them.

4.2.4 Participatory Governance: Multi-Stakeholder Engagement Beyond Expert Domination

Participatory governance creates formal structures that embed the voices of users, communities, and frontline actors in shaping behavioral health systems. It addresses a long-standing governance failure: the systemic exclusion of those most affected from the decisions that define access, safety, and care delivery.

Traditional governance in behavioral health has privileged professional and institutional perspectives, often sidelining those with lived experience. This imbalance has produced systems that are technically robust but misaligned with real-world needs—eroding trust, relevance, and cultural responsiveness.

Participatory governance reconfigures this dynamic through:

- **Multi-stakeholder governance bodies** → Formal structures that include users, caregivers, clinicians, and implementers in decision-making
- **Lived experience integration** → Mechanisms for incorporating first-hand insight into policy design, implementation, and evaluation

- **Decision transparency** → Public visibility into how choices are made, whose interests are represented, and what feedback loops exist

This model aligns with WHO Modules 1 and 2, which call for the integration of people with lived experience into system design and monitoring (World Health Organization, 2025a, 2025b). The 5P Model operationalizes this principle at scale—moving participation from a value statement to a structural governance function embedded within digital ecosystems.

Governance Insight
Participation must be designed as a system function, not an advisory add-on. Governance legitimacy depends on the inclusion of those subject to its decisions—not only for justice but for real-world effectiveness.

While digital tools increasingly promote "patient-centered" care through data access and personal dashboards, access alone does not constitute empowerment. In behavioral health—where stigma, diagnostic ambiguity, and emotional vulnerability intersect—data transparency without interpretive support can amplify confusion, anxiety, or self-blame. Without cultural grounding or epistemic scaffolding, participation risks becoming an illusion: a shift of responsibility without a redistribution of knowledge or power.

Participatory governance must therefore move beyond the rhetoric of inclusion. It must create collective epistemologies, ensure training and interpretability, and protect against the privatization of risk through individualized data delivery.

Still, inclusion alone is not enough. Governance must also respond proportionally to risk—ensuring that precision, not uniformity, defines oversight. This is the aim of precise governance.

4.2.5 Precision Governance

Precision governance calibrates oversight according to specific risk profiles, implementation contexts, and levels of evidence—moving beyond one-size-fits-all approaches that can either stifle innovation or fail to address serious risks. In digital behavioral health, where interventions range from mood trackers to predictive diagnostic tools, precision is not optional—it is a governance imperative.

Traditional regulatory systems apply uniform requirements regardless of clinical risk, user group, or technological complexity. This creates a paradox: low-risk tools face disproportionate barriers, while high-risk algorithms may evade meaningful scrutiny. In environments defined by dynamic, distributed, and user-driven interventions, *blunt regulatory instruments are structurally inadequate*.

Precision governance reconfigures oversight through:

- **Risk-calibrated frameworks** → Requirements scale with potential harm, use case, and technological complexity.
- **Evidence-proportionate regulation** → The strength of evidence reflects the claims and context of each system.
- **Implementation-sensitive standards** → Oversight adapts to real-world variability, deployment setting, and user diversity.

In essence, precision governance recognizes that not all digital mental health technologies represent the same level of risk or require the same level of oversight. While a simple mood tracking app may need light-touch regulation, a predictive diagnostic algorithm using artificial intelligence demands much more rigorous scrutiny. The aim is to create a governance framework flexible enough not to stifle innovation but robust enough to effectively protect users.

This precision is not simply about optimizing approval—it is an ethical safeguard. As Adler et al. (2022a, 2022b) demonstrate, machine learning models for digital mental health biomarkers often perform well in controlled environments but collapse across demographic groups, timeframes, or device types. Without governance mechanisms that enforce population-equitable validation, systems risk entrenching bias under the illusion of objectivity.

Building on this insight, Nordberg et al. (2024) uncovered another significant governance gap in digital mental health technologies. Even highly sophisticated sensing models designed to forecast adolescent mental health deterioration—which promise unprecedented early intervention capabilities—often lack critical standards for implementation, interpretability, and clinical oversight. These systems may operate with impressive behavioral depth, but their lack of comprehensive accountability creates what the researchers term a risk of "precision without protection."

This accountability challenge extends beyond predictive models. Youn et al. (2025) revealed how the absence of robust governance mechanisms can transform potentially supportive digital tools into sources of professional burden. Their research demonstrated that clinical decision support tools, when deployed without nuanced, risk-tiered governance or contextual feedback loops, can paradoxically increase cognitive and ethical strain for frontline healthcare providers. What Nordberg's team identified as a technical precision problem, Youn's research exposed as a practical implementation crisis—both pointing to the urgent need for more sophisticated, context-aware governance frameworks.

Emerging frameworks like Germany's *DiGA model* illustrate the potential of performance-based regulation. Yet certification alone is insufficient. Precision governance requires a *hybrid ecosystem* where clinical logic, technical standards, public health needs, and participatory input align.

Governance Insight

Precision must be more than a technical virtue—it must be a structural logic that ensures oversight remains equitable, proportional, and relevant in fast-evolving systems.

But even precisely calibrated systems can fail if they wait for harm to appear. In digital behavioral health, the real opportunity lies upstream—in governing systems that intervene before breakdown. This is the logic of preventive governance.

Integrating the 5P Governance Mechanisms

Together, these five governance mechanisms address the core challenges that arise when behavioral health systems shift from workforce-centered to data-centered operation. The 5P Model provides not just technical scaffolding but a redefinition of governance itself, rooted in anticipatory design, ethical accountability, and systemic coherence.

Crucially, the 5P Model is not something to be "implemented" solely in hospitals or health centers. It must guide how ministries of health write policy, how funders assess value, how health professionals are trained, and how digital platforms are held accountable for the tools they release. In this way, the model operates simultaneously across three levels:

1. **Clinical care**—guiding therapeutic strategies and patient engagement
2. **Systemic design**—informing how systems fund, train, and structure services
3. **Governance and ethics**—shaping law, regulation, and global equity agendas

The strength of the 5P approach lies not only in what it enables but in what it displaces: time-bound reimbursement, symptom-only diagnostics, national silos, and rigid professional hierarchies. Displacing these outdated models is essential to build behavioral health systems that are effective, equitable, and future ready.

4.2.6 From Evidence to Accountability: Diagnosing the Governance Gap

Systematic reviews of digital behavioral health governance have identified patterns of success across diverse implementations that align with the 5P framework. Meta-analyses by Torous et al. (2021), examining over 120 digital mental health initiatives, found that governance integration across predictive, preventive, personalized, participatory, and precision-based dimensions was associated with significantly higher implementation success rates and sustained outcomes. Similarly, the WHO's global review of digital mental health frameworks (2023) highlighted that coordinated governance mechanisms were critical success factors across 18 national implementation programs.

Multiple implementation studies reinforce this pattern. Germany's DiGA program demonstrated the effectiveness of precision-based and participatory governance in improving regulatory efficiency while maintaining clinical standards (Schmidt et al., 2023). Singapore's population-level early detection systems exemplify predictive and preventive governance through integrated technical and clinical oversight. Cross-border initiatives like the WHO's Step-by-Step program show how personalized governance can adapt frameworks to diverse cultural contexts while maintaining core standards.

Recent frameworks underscore that the challenge is not only *whether* governance exists but *how* it aligns across sociotechnical layers. Pourat et al. (2022), in evaluating behavioral health integration across US systems, found that while infrastructure maturity scored relatively high, care coordination and referral processes lagged—highlighting a persistent fragmentation between system design and delivery. This disconnect is not merely operational; it reveals a structural governance breakdown. Meanwhile, Malgaroli et al. (2025) propose a sociocultural–technical framework for large language models (LLMs) in mental health, emphasizing that responsible AI use demands more than technical safeguards: it requires inclusive development processes, culturally sensitive design, and governance mechanisms that translate code into care. These frameworks highlight the structural necessity of roles capable of bridging clinical, technical, and ethical governance domains.

These findings align with broader implementation research. As Mohr et al. (2025) note, "The primary barriers to effective digital behavioral health implementation were not technological but related to governance translation across disciplinary boundaries." This cross-domain governance gap has emerged as a structural limitation that transcends individual professional capabilities.

In this context, barriers to full implementation of the 5P Model include:

- Resistance from legacy institutions and credentialing boards unprepared for cross-domain roles
- Fragmented funding models that do not account for governance functions
- Lack of operational metrics to assess governance effectiveness
- Jurisdictional ambiguity over responsibility for oversight in hybrid, AI-mediated systems
- Weak pathways for training and certifying governance-specific professionals

These barriers point to a deeper challenge: digital behavioral health cannot be governed effectively without redefining responsibility. It is not merely a question of data or design but of who is accountable, across what layers, and under what logic.

Reconnecting the Governance Chain
The 5P Model introduces a new logic of distributed, anticipatory governance. But without clear accountability mechanisms, it risks replicating the same gaps it seeks to solve.

4.2 The 5P Components as Governance Mechanisms

Table 4.2 Governance accountability in the 5P Model

5P function	Who pays?	Who benefits?	Who governs?	Who is accountable?	5P governance fix
Predictive	Public systems, insurers, investors	Tech firms (data assets), platforms, populations (if governed)	Algorithms (opaque), tech firms	No one clearly—harm discovered late	Embed predictive systems into regulated public infrastructure with validation and clinical logic
Preventive	Governments, employers, platforms	Employers (reduced costs), users, platforms (engagement)	App developers, behavioral scientists	Fragmented: no thresholds or standards	Define ethical triggers, thresholds, and recourse mechanisms
Personalized	Donors, ministries, philanthropy	Marginalized populations, health equity agendas	Often ignored or underfunded	Exclusion persists	Fund adaptive governance to replace one-size-fits-all standards
Participatory	Public grants, health systems	Users, communities, civil society	Rarely formalized	Symbolic inclusion without power	Build multi-stakeholder governance bodies with formal authority
Precision	Regulators, platforms, compliance investors	Developers (fast approval), users (if valid)	Regulatory bodies (often under-resourced)	Limited: over- or under-regulated	Enforce risk-calibrated, context-sensitive standards with real-world testing

Table 4.2 presents a comprehensive realignment framework. It synthesizes the full governance logic of the 5P Model—not just who pays but who benefits, who governs, and who is accountable. This is the broken chain the model aims to repair.

This table is not a best practice checklist—it is a diagnostic and realignment tool. It enables governments, funders, and institutions to clarify who pays, who benefits, who governs, who is accountable, and how systems can be designed to prevent harm before it occurs.

Crucially, these gaps are not only technical or ethical—they are economic. As discussed in Chap. 2, mental health systems are shaped by fragmented funding, misaligned incentives, and shallow accountability structures that undermine long-term value. Without governance mechanisms that align investment with real value creation, digital tools risk amplifying rather than addressing systemic inequities.

Chapter 5 returns to this challenge, reframing value governance as a core implementation function.

The 5P framework gains traction only when embedded in a concrete accountability ecosystem. As such, the final barrier to implementation is conceptual: understanding governance not as a constraint on innovation but as its precondition. Systems that scale without governance do not scale ethically. They scale risk, inequity, and opacity.

Conclusion Linkage: From Diagnostic to Design
This framework is not the conclusion but the pivot point toward operational design. The logic of accountability must now be translated into roles and capacities.

This transition demands a new type of professional capable of translating governance diagnostics into design—anticipating, coordinating, and sustaining ethical infrastructures. This is the work of the Digital Behavioral Health Expert (DBHE). Section 4.3 explores this role in detail.

4.3 The Digital Behavioral Health Expert: A Governance Catalyst

The implementation of the 5P governance framework requires more than institutional alignment—it demands a new kind of professional equipped to operate across clinical, technical, and regulatory boundaries. The Digital Behavioral Health Expert (DBHE) emerges as this governance catalyst: a role specifically designed to embed,

Table 4.3 Strategic and operational levels in digital behavioral health governance

Governance level	Professional profile	Role description	Example responsibilities
Strategic governance	Digital behavioral health expert (DBHE)	Managerial oversight, coordination of policy, ethical frameworks, and systemic integration	Establishing governance frameworks, overseeing algorithmic transparency, coordinating stakeholder engagement, shaping regulatory adaptation
Operational implementation	Behavioral health technician	Direct integration and management of digital tools within care environments, ensuring compliance with DBHE-set guidelines	Implementing digital interventions, managing patient data and consent processes, monitoring daily algorithmic operations, escalating compliance concerns to DBHE

This table distinguishes between the strategic governance role of the DBHE and the operational functions of behavioral health technicians. It illustrates how the 5P Model translates into workforce roles across levels of responsibility. Detailed implementation strategies and training pathways are provided in Chap. 5

4.3 The Digital Behavioral Health Expert: A Governance Catalyst

translate, and sustain the 5P logic within systems that increasingly operate beyond the reach of traditional professional mediation.

This profile builds upon the foundational vision introduced in Ethics in Digital Mental Health (Martí Noguera, 2024), where Chap. 7 outlined the ethical competencies of the Digital Behavioral Health Expert. That chapter emphasized the imperative of cultivating ethically grounded capacity to manage AI, supervise data-driven tools, and preserve the therapeutic alliance within increasingly hybrid ecosystems. These ethical foundations—centered on human-AI collaboration, interpretability, data protection, and algorithmic oversight—remain essential to the DBHE profile.

However, this chapter extends that foundation into a full-spectrum governance architecture. The DBHE is not merely an ethically aware clinician or technician—it is a cross-domain professional trained to coordinate data governance, evaluate algorithms, apply implementation science, and navigate policy environments. This evolution responds to the growing complexity of digital ecosystems and to the urgent need for *operational governance roles* that go beyond ethical awareness to enable systemic accountability.

Table 4.3 introduces the distinction between these strategic and operational roles, providing clarity that will be further expanded and operationalized with practical implementation details in Chap. 5. This structured differentiation aligns workforce development strategies with the growing complexity of digital ecosystems and the critical need for comprehensive governance in digital behavioral health.

> **Important: Core Competencies Rooted in Ethics**
>
> The competencies defined in *Ethics in Digital Mental Health* (Martí Noguera, 2024)—particularly around human-AI collaboration, supervision of digital systems, data integrity, and the ethical management of emerging technologies—remain foundational to the DBHE role. Section 4.3 builds on this ethical foundation and integrates it into a governance-ready operational profile for digital behavioral health systems.
>
> While the WHO's workforce development directives (Module 2) highlight the need for expanded roles and new competencies in mental health systems (World Health Organization, 2025b), they stop short of defining digital governance capabilities. The *DBHE fills this critical gap*—bridging the WHO's policy vision with the operational realities of hybrid, AI-enabled, and data-driven care ecosystems.

4.3.1 Strategic Rationale for the DBHE: Bridging Systems in Transition

Current healthcare governance faces a critical structural gap between evolving digital infrastructure and the professional capacity required to govern it. While clinicians, technologists, and regulators each possess essential domain knowledge, few professionals are equipped to navigate the complex intersections between these domains—particularly in behavioral health systems increasingly mediated by data, algorithms, and distributed care models.

As detailed in Chap. 1, the shift from territorial, state-bound governance to transnational, platform-mediated ecosystems has fundamentally redefined what it means to "govern" behavioral health. While governments and health systems have made bold digital investments—AI strategies, telehealth infrastructures, and national data policies—most lack the human infrastructure to implement these technologies with ethical and systemic oversight.

This section marks a strategic inflection point: moving from analysis to action. The table below synthesizes global cases that illustrate this challenge. On the one side is sophisticated digital strategies, and on the other is insufficient cross-domain governance capacity. This gap is precisely what the 5P governance model—and the DBHE role—seeks to address.

As illustrated in Table 4.4, this structural misalignment between advanced digital strategies and specialized governance workforce is evident across diverse global

Table 4.4 Digital mental health strategies vs. workforce preparedness

Region	Digital health strategy	Mental health digitalization	Specialized workforce (DBHE)	Identified gap
European Union	EHDS, DECODE, AI Act	High (EHRs, mental health apps, ethical frameworks)	Emerging (digital skills; no dedicated DBHE roles)	Lack of cross-cutting competencies for behavioral health governance
United states	NIH/NIMH Playbooks, ONC Health IT, VA Connected Care	Medium-high (telepsychiatry, digital CBT, integration)	Fragmented (IT, clinicians, admins; no unified role)	Siloed roles; absence of governance mediators across technical and clinical fields
Singapore	Smart Nation, HealthTech Masterplan	High (AI-driven early detection, centralized systems)	Partial (integrated leadership roles)	Gaps in ethical-regulatory alignment
Saudi Arabia	Vision 2030, Seha Virtual Hospital, National Mental Health Strategy	Medium (national coverage, emerging digital pathways)	Low (limited digital capacity in mental health)	Need for hybrid governance profiles
China	National Digital Health Strategy, AI-powered community systems (Tree Hole, MentalBERT)	High (AI, NLP, population-wide deployment)	Partial (technical AI roles; clinical link missing)	Risks of overreach without cross-domain oversight

4.3 The Digital Behavioral Health Expert: A Governance Catalyst

regions, highlighting the urgent need for professionals capable of bridging these domains. This domain gap manifests in governance failures including:

- Privacy breaches due to inadequate data governance
- Implementation failures from poor integration into clinical workflows
- Equity gaps when digital tools are designed without inclusive stakeholder input
- Regulatory inconsistencies that either stifle innovation or fail to protect users

These failures are not technical oversights—they are governance gaps. As systems transition from workforce-centered to data-centered operation, the DBHE becomes essential infrastructure to ensure that digital health transformation remains accountable, equitable, and effective.

4.3.2 Essential Competencies for Cross-Domain Governance

The DBHE represents a professional profile specifically designed to bridge the governance gap between clinical and technical domains. Unlike clinical specialists focused on treatment or technical developers focused on tool creation, the DBHE operates within a distinct governance layer—ensuring the ethical, equitable, and effective integration of digital systems into behavioral health ecosystems.

This approach aligns with a growing international consensus on the need for governance-oriented digital competencies. For instance, the DECODE framework (Car et al., 2025), developed under the EU4Health Programme, outlines interdisciplinary, ethics-driven competencies required for digital transformation. Similarly, Brommeyer et al. (2023) highlight that most postgraduate health management programs fail to address over half of the digital leadership competencies needed in future health systems—especially in behavioral health. Holland Brown and Bewick (2022) add that UK healthcare professionals often lack formal digital health education and instead rely on anecdotal sources or consumer app ratings—posing systemic governance risks. Likewise, Pote et al. (2021) examined clinical psychology doctoral programs in the United Kingdom and found that only 3 of 18 institutions offered formal training in digital mental health competencies. Their findings highlighted barriers such as curriculum inertia, faculty capacity, and infrastructure limitations—factors that delay the integration of digital governance into clinical education.

Several of the competencies defined in *Ethics in Digital Mental Health* (Martí Noguera, 2024) remain directly relevant here. These include the supervision of AI systems and clinical data, development of collaborative relationships with AI, and ethical management of sensitive data—competencies that now underpin DBHE practice.

Core governance competencies of the DBHE include:

- Data governance expertise → Designing frameworks for responsible data collection, sharing, and accountability
- Algorithm evaluation skills → Identifying bias, drift, and usability issues in digital tools that influence behavioral health outcomes
- Implementation science knowledge → Understanding what enables or blocks integration into care workflows and training environments

- Policy navigation capabilities → Interpreting, applying, and shaping relevant legal and ethical guidelines across jurisdictions
- Stakeholder engagement abilities → Building inclusive, multi-stakeholder processes that anchor governance in real-world diversity

These competencies enable the DBHE to:

- Translate between clinical, technical, and regulatory languages
- Identify and remediate governance gaps across systems
- Coordinate implementation of oversight frameworks at scale
- Monitor digital ecosystems to guide iterative system improvement

In this way, the DBHE ensures that governance is not reduced to compliance but becomes a continuous, collaborative function embedded across digital behavioral health systems. These validated competencies form the foundation for DBHE implementation, workforce development, and system integration strategies—detailed in Chap. 5.

4.3.3 Knowledge Translation Between Regulatory Frameworks and Implementation Contexts

The Digital Behavioral Health Expert (DBHE) plays a pivotal role in translating abstract governance principles into actionable, context-sensitive systems. Unlike traditional compliance officers who interpret regulation through a binary lens of adherence, the DBHE engages in continuous translation—where ethical frameworks, clinical realities, and technical systems converge.

This translation is neither symbolic nor static. It is a dynamic, bidirectional function that adapts global governance mandates to local realities while feeding frontline insights back into policy discourse. In behavioral health, where stigma, platform variation, and uneven data quality converge, such translation becomes an ethical act of stewardship.

The DBHE enacts this role across three interconnected domains:

- Contextual adaptation → Mapping governance values (equity, accountability, transparency) onto specific operational realities—whether that be a public health chatbot in Singapore or a private therapy app in Alberta
- Bidirectional learning → Using feedback from implementation to inform the design of future tools, standards, and interventions—thereby anchoring governance in lived practice
- Ethical alignment → Ensuring that oversight structures protect user rights, therapeutic relationships, and contextual fairness—not just institutional liability

Context in Flux: Canada's AI Governance Gap
Recent developments in Canada underscore the fragility of governance translation. With the 2025 prorogation of Parliament, critical legislation like Bill C-27—intended to modernize PIPEDA and introduce the Artificial Intelligence and Data

4.3 The Digital Behavioral Health Expert: A Governance Catalyst   69

Table 4.5 Translating governance dimensions: functions and examples across regions

Dimension	Translation function	Example
Regulatory to operational	Adapting national or international frameworks to local workflows and platform architectures	EU Cross-Border eHealth Services integrated privacy-by-design protocols through DBHE-led translation of GDPR and AI Act requirements[a]
Implementation to policy	Feeding real-world data, failures, and friction points back into governance design	India's Tele-MANAS system integrates frontline feedback on digital mental health helplines to inform centralized standards and escalation policies[b]
Ethical to technical	Embedding patient safety, transparency, and fairness into system features	DBHE roles in Singapore's Smart Health Clinics ensure risk-tiered triage systems respect cultural and privacy expectations[c]

[a] European Commission (2022)
[b] Government of India (2022)
[c] Singapore MOH (2023)

Act (AIDA)—has stalled. As of early 2025, no comprehensive national AI regulation is in place. This leaves behavioral health systems navigating AI deployment with outdated privacy laws and no clear framework for algorithmic accountability. The DBHE becomes essential in this vacuum: translating ethical best practices, ensuring user protection, and contextualizing platform risks even in the absence of legislative clarity.

Governance Insight
Translation is not interpretation—it is operationalization. A DBHE does not merely "apply" rules. They reconcile intent with reality, ethics with scalability, and regulatory gaps with anticipatory design.

This is where governance shifts from theory to practice and where the DBHE becomes the anchor of responsible digital behavioral health implementation.

Table 4.5 summarizes the translation dimensions.

4.3.4 *Enabling Governance in Environments of Diminishing Professional Mediation*

As digital behavioral health systems evolve, a growing share of clinical decisions, triage processes, and therapeutic nudges occurs without direct professional oversight. Instead, these interactions are mediated by algorithms, behavioral data flows, and platform architectures—shifting the operational locus of care from human expertise to system logic.

In this emerging paradigm, governance must evolve beyond professional proximity. Traditional safeguards—rooted in licensure, human supervision, or institutional ethics boards—become insufficient in contexts where millions of user interactions unfold continuously, asynchronously, and often invisibly.

The DBHE plays a central role in enabling governance in these environments by designing, operationalizing, and monitoring mechanisms that uphold ethical integrity and system accountability—despite the decreasing presence of professionals at the point of care.

Key governance functions in low-mediation environments include:

- Establishing algorithmic governance frameworks → Ensuring that digital systems used for triage, symptom monitoring, or recommendation have built-in transparency, bias detection, and ethical guardrails
- Developing oversight mechanisms for data-centered care → Creating dashboards, escalation protocols, and audit trails that allow for indirect but effective professional and institutional supervision
- Anticipating emergent risks → Identifying governance blind spots that may arise not from isolated failures but from systemic design patterns (e.g., feedback loops that reinforce inequity)
- Embedding safeguards into system design → Collaborating with developers and regulators to embed safety features that do not depend on human intervention—such as differential privacy layers, user agency prompts, or automated consent refreshers

This shift does not imply abandoning clinical expertise but repositioning it. In environments of diminishing professional mediation, the role of the DBHE is to re-institutionalize governance: embedding professional values into system logic, ensuring mechanisms exist for course correction, and reinforcing the rights and safety of users who may never meet a clinician.

- Case Example: Singapore's AI-Mediated Early Detection
  In Singapore's Smart Nation mental health initiative, early detection of distress is increasingly driven by population-level behavioral data rather than direct professional assessment. DBHEs have been instrumental in developing governance protocols that ensure triage decisions made by AI systems remain interpretable, risk tiered, and ethically aligned—ensuring population scale does not come at the cost of individual protection (Singapore MOH, 2023).
- Governance Insight
  In data-centered systems, the absence of professional mediation must not mean the absence of professional judgment. The DBHE ensures that human values are not removed but translated, encoded, and monitored through governance architectures designed for scale.
- Transition Note
  While this chapter has focused on the strategic rationale, core competencies, and governance functions of the DBHE, the practical question of how to train, credential, and integrate this profile across diverse systems requires dedicated attention. Chapter 5 will explore these implementation pathways—translating vision into workforce development strategies at scale.

4.4 Ethical Governance Across Systems: From Fragmented Roles to the DBHE Logic

As governments partner with technology sectors to expand access to mental healthcare, digital behavioral health is transitioning from fragmented pilot programs to national infrastructures. These global investments reflect a growing recognition that mental health must be accessible, scalable, and ethically governed. Yet these efforts raise difficult questions about oversight, equity, and responsibility.

This section reframes implementation cases not as isolated examples but as illustrations of ethical tensions in digital behavioral health governance and how the Digital Behavioral Health Expert (DBHE) can enable systems to respond responsibly, equitably, and at scale. As behavioral health becomes increasingly mediated by data and platforms, ethics must move from advisory statements to embedded system functions.

This evolution is not only technical—it is ethical and professional. As outlined in Sect. 3.5, clinician literacy and legacy governance models are often too slow to adapt. The 5P framework thus evolves from a conceptual model into a borderless, practice-oriented architecture where DBHE roles emerge to institutionalize governance capacities in increasingly hybrid and transnational systems.

The following cases demonstrate how the 5P governance framework supports ethical governance functions when operationalized through the DBHE role. Rather than offer descriptive summaries, we analyze governance gaps, professional implications, and institutional needs.

- From program design to governance capacity, what unites the diverse implementations analyzed in this section?

    - Digital behavioral health is outpacing traditional governance → Clinical and ethical oversight is increasingly distributed across AI systems, apps, and platforms.
    - Ethical tensions arise from structural gaps → These include lack of professional roles, unclear responsibility for harms, and fragmented regulatory tools.
    - Legacy roles (clinician, regulator, technologist) cannot alone ensure ethical implementation → Silos create blind spots.
    - The DBHE addresses this convergence → Enabling cross-domain negotiation, ethical adaptation, and oversight in complex, hybrid environments.
    - The 5P Model evolves with practice → It moves from a normative framework to a governance architecture adaptable to national and cross-border implementation.

These insights justify a shift from case-by-case digital solutions to embedded governance capacity. The DBHE is not a stopgap—it is the infrastructure for making digital behavioral health systems ethically operable.

> Ethical governance is not only about guidelines—it requires professionals capable of recognizing, negotiating, and institutionalizing governance functions across clinical, technical, and regulatory domains. The DBHE plays a pivotal role in making ethical governance actionable in real-world systems. As Stroud et al. (2025) note, "Although these harms may be more abstract than direct risks to individuals, their potential impacts remain relevant and warrant ethical consideration."

Governance at Scale Beyond Professional Mediation (India)—India's Tele-MANAS demonstrates how digital behavioral health can scale ethically without traditional workforce expansion. Tiered services integrate human and digital supports, offering multilingual, culturally adapted access points (Government of India, 2022; WHO, 2024).

Ethical Tension → Can equitable, culturally relevant care be scaled without compromising safety or inclusion?
DBHE Function → Operationalizing oversight in local adaptation, algorithmic fairness, and escalation thresholds.
5P Dimensions → Predictive, personalized, participatory, precise, and preventive.
Insight → Systems can scale ethically, but without defined governance roles like the DBHE, oversight remains ad hoc and fragile.

Balancing Innovation and Protection The DiGA Model (Germany)—Germany's DiGA program integrates mental health apps into statutory healthcare with structured evaluation and reimbursement (BfArM, 2023; Arcà et al., 2025).

Ethical Tension → How can systems balance speed of innovation with meaningful accountability?
DBHE Function → Supporting evidence interpretation, bias assessment, and stakeholder engagement.
5P Dimensions → Personalized, precise, and participative.
Insight → Even advanced regulatory models need governance translation at the local level—underscoring the DBHE's role in navigating use contexts.

Cross-Border Governance Step-by-Step (WHO)—The WHO's Step-by-Step app operates across displaced and conflict-affected populations with culturally adapted self-help tools (WHO, 2022).

Ethical Tension → How can governance ensure clinical integrity and user protection in fractured jurisdictions?
DBHE Function → Translating global standards into local contexts and feeding user data back into iterative design.
5P Dimensions → Predictive, personalized, and participatory.
Insight → The DBHE is vital in fragile settings to embed ethics in systems that may lack regulatory infrastructure.

4.4 Ethical Governance Across Systems: From Fragmented Roles to the DBHE Logic

- **Case Box: Qatar's WMHQ and Cultural Fit in Global Frameworks**
  Qatar's World Mental Health Qatar (WMHQ) study demonstrates how global research protocols can integrate culturally responsive governance. By aligning neuroimaging and clinical assessment tools with local social norms, WMHQ reframed international standards to fit regional realities (Khaled et al., 2024).
  DBHE Insight → In culturally sensitive implementations, the DBHE mediates between global epistemologies and local legitimacy—ensuring governance does not merely transfer models but co-constructs relevance.

- **Case Box: Comparing Early Detection Logics—Singapore vs. United States**
  Singapore's national strategy integrates AI-powered behavioral analytics to anticipate distress in schools, workplaces, and communities. This approach redefines early detection as a population-level triage system—where predictive governance becomes a core function of public health infrastructure (Singapore MOH, 2023).
  In contrast, the US implementation described by Youn et al. (2025) embeds early detection directly into clinical workflows, aligning it with existing provider practices and minimizing disruption.
  DBHE Insight → These systems reflect distinct operational logics: one preclinical and algorithmic and the other clinical and relational. Both require governance roles capable of aligning predictive tools with ethical safeguards and user trust.

- **Case Box: Co-creation and Cultural Governance in China**
  Sit et al. (2024) propose a five-stage digital mental health implementation model in China that integrates co-creation, cultural adaptation, and iterative governance evaluation. It begins with expert consultations and culminates in sustainable, context-aware delivery—addressing not just technical feasibility but cultural legitimacy.
  DBHE Insight → The DBHE plays a pivotal role in sustaining this governance loop—ensuring that cultural adaptations are institutionalized, not episodic, and that user realities inform each design and oversight layer.

Governance and Equity Ethical and Economic Frontiers—Global implementations reveal that governance gaps often stem not from technical deficits but from underdeveloped economic and ethical design.

Ethical Tension → How can systems avoid reproducing inequity through underinvestment, misaligned incentives, or privacy overreach?
DBHE Function → Reframing value and ensuring economic governance aligns with ethical care delivery.
Cases → UK's IAPT (NHS England, 2023), Singapore (Singapore MOH, 2023), Saudi Arabia (Almubarak & Alhabeeb, 2024), Australia (Australian Commission on Safety and Quality in Health Care, 2023), China (Huang & Hu, 2024).
5P Dimensions → All five dimensions variably expressed.
Insight → Ethical and economic governance must converge, and the DBHE is critical in mediating this convergence across systems.

This framing also echoes Stroud et al.'s (2025) cautionary insight: "We do not offer these suggestions as best practices... but as one AMC's efforts to develop AI governance strategies in the absence of clear regulatory policies and guidelines." Their experience underscores why the DBHE role is essential—not to enforce static best practices but to continuously negotiate ethical governance in evolving, ambiguous environments.

These cases make clear that digital ethics cannot remain abstract—they must be enacted through embedded roles like the DBHE. Chapter 5 builds on this foundation by exploring how ethical oversight becomes a formalized, trainable, and scalable workforce function. It presents implementation strategies to build governance capacity, ensure workforce readiness, and design institutions that align with the 5P Model.

4.5 Conclusion: Governance as Transformation Catalyst

The 5P Model fundamentally reframes digital behavioral health transformation as a governance challenge rather than merely a technological one—echoing foundational critiques from Chap. 1 on professional workforce constraints and Chap. 2's analysis of economic governance misalignments. As shown in Chap. 3, the 5P framework grew out of the need to bridge normative ambition with implementable logic, and here it is reconfirmed as the structural anchor for ethically sound, data-centered systems operating across borders and platforms. As the preceding cases show, ethical oversight, institutional coordination, and equity require more than tools—they demand embedded governance capacity. In a landscape increasingly defined by AI-driven decisions, cross-border platforms, and asynchronous care models, the model offers not a framework for evaluation but a logic for ethical implementation.

Each component of the model—predictive, personalized, participatory, precise, and preventive—addresses governance challenges that emerge in the transition from workforce-centered to data-centered systems. But as digital behavioral health expands, the 5P Model evolves as well. What began as a normative model now operates as a governance architecture—adaptable to diverse contexts and capable of institutional translation through roles like the Digital Behavioral Health Expert (DBHE).

The DBHE has emerged across this chapter not as a theoretical actor but as a response to urgent system needs: from managing ethical risks in data flows, to translating global standards into local contexts, to navigating economic misalignments and surveillance dilemmas. Implementation examples from Germany, India, Singapore, Australia, Qatar, China, Rwanda, the United Kingdom, Saudi Arabia, and the United States (including the case study by Youn et al., 2025) illustrate the real-world relevance of the DBHE and 5P governance framework. As detailed in Sect. 4.4, these cases highlight diverse cultural and regulatory contexts, yet all converge around one insight: that effective digital behavioral health systems require embedded governance, not just digital capacity. This empirical foundation strengthens the model's credibility and affirms its flexibility across geographies and resource levels.

4.5 Conclusion: Governance as Transformation Catalyst

This chapter's reframing of implementation—from case-by-case to ethical convergence—shows that digital behavioral health is not facing a tech gap but a governance capacity gap. Ethical governance is not achieved through guidelines alone; it requires new professional infrastructure and cross-system coherence.

The DBHE addresses this challenge by:

- Bridging regulatory, clinical, and technical domains
- Operationalizing the 5P logic at scale
- Anchoring ethical principles in system design, not just documentation

Metrics Beyond Time-Based Care

To close this chapter, we turn to one of the most persistent governance bottlenecks: how we measure success. This section is a continuation of the conclusion, highlighting operational priorities rather than introducing a new thematic block.

Current healthcare systems remain governed by metrics such as billable hours, session counts, or inpatient days—proxies of professional effort rather than system performance. This legacy reflects not only entrenched reimbursement logic but also a deep dependency on professional mediation. As discussed in Chap. 1, such metrics presuppose stable clinical workflows and abundant workforce capacity—conditions no longer viable in data-centered systems operating at scale.

The 5P Model demands a shift toward outcome-oriented, longitudinal metrics that reflect engagement, adaptability, and social reintegration. Predictive prevention, for example, should be rewarded for avoiding escalation—not penalized for reducing clinic visits. This insight aligns with Chap. 2's critique of value-based care models that fail to capture digital-era dynamics and often reinforce institutional inertia.

An evaluation of public hospitals in California underscores this challenge.

Additionally, large-scale behavioral economics initiatives in wellness promotion demonstrate how long-term, incentive-driven behavior change frameworks can shape engagement. Though not always framed explicitly as mental health governance, these programs highlight how predictive, precise, and participatory strategies can generate longitudinal engagement—a principle essential to the 5P logic.

Without these instruments, health systems risk defaulting to outdated, time-based metrics that obscure what truly matters: early intervention, user engagement, contextual adaptability, and long-term outcomes.

Looking forward, the 5P Model offers a roadmap for aligning normative aspirations with implementation realities. It supports policymakers, healthcare leaders, and technology developers in building systems that are technically effective and ethically legitimate.

The next chapter builds directly on the operational and ethical groundwork laid in Chap. 4. It moves from governance vision to implementation strategy, offering a structured playbook for translating the 5P Model into actionable, system-wide change. By operationalizing the principles discussed here, Chap. 5 guides policymakers, developers, and clinical leaders through the transition from conceptual governance to institutional transformation. It presents a playbook for applying the 5P framework across organizational, regional, and national systems—turning ethical design into institutional transformation and measurable impact.

References

Adams, J. (2024). Examining ethical and social implications of digital mental health technologies through expert interviews and sociotechnical systems theory. *DISO, 3*, 24. https://doi.org/10.1007/s44206-024-00110-5

Adil, M., Atiq, I., & Younus, S. (2024). Effectiveness of the apple watch as a mental health tracker. *Journal of Global Health, 14*, 03010. https://doi.org/10.7189/jogh.14.03010

Adler, D. A., Wang, F., Mohr, D. C., & Choudhury, T. (2022a). Machine learning for passive mental health symptom prediction: Generalization across different longitudinal mobile sensing studies. *PLoS One, 17*(4), e0266516. https://doi.org/10.1371/journal.pone.0266516

Adler DA, Wang F, Mohr DC, Estrin D, Livesey C, Choudhury T (2022b) A call for open data to develop mental health digital biomarkers. BJPsych Open 8(2):e58. https://doi.org/10.1192/bjo.2022.28.

Aksunger, N., Vernot, C., Littman, R., Voors, M., Meriggi, N. F., Abajobir, A., Beber, B., Dai, K., Egger, D., Islam, A., Kelly, J., Kharel, A., Matabaro, A., Moya, A., Mwachofi, P., Nekesa, C., Ochieng, E., Rahman, T., Scacco, A., van Dalen, Y., et al. (2023). COVID-19 and mental health in 8 low- and middle-income countries: A prospective cohort study. *PLoS Medicine, 20*(4), e1004081. https://doi.org/10.1371/journal.pmed.1004081

Al Dweik, R., Ajaj, R., Kotb, R., et al. (2024). Opportunities and challenges in leveraging digital technology for mental health system strengthening: A systematic review to inform interventions in The United Arab Emirates. *BMC Public Health, 24*, 2592. https://doi.org/10.1186/s12889-024-19980-y

Almubarak, L. N., & Alhabeeb, A. A. (2024). The mental health system in the Kingdom of Saudi Arabia. *Journal of Biomedical Research & Environmental Sciences, 5*(7), 773–778. https://doi.org/10.37871/jbres1954

Arcà, E., Heldt, D., & Smith, M. (2025). Comparison of health technology assessments for digital therapeutics in Germany, the United Kingdom and France. *Digital Health, 11*, 1–14. https://doi.org/10.1177/20552076241308704

Australian Commission on Safety and Quality in Health Care. (2023). *National safety and quality digital mental health standards*. ACSQHC.

Bednarz, Z., Lewis, K., & Sadowski, J. (2024). It's not personal, it's strictly business: Behavioural insurance and the impacts of non-personal data on individuals, groups and societies. *Computer Law & Security Review, 54*, 106096. https://doi.org/10.1016/j.clsr.2024.106096

Bennett-Levy, J., Singer, J., Rotumah, D., Bernays, S., & Edwards, D. (2021). From Digital Mental Health to Digital Social and Emotional Wellbeing: How Indigenous Community-Based Participatory Research Influenced the Australian Government's Digital Mental Health Agenda. *International Journal of Environmental Research and Public Health, 18*(18), 9757. https://doi.org/10.3390/ijerph18189757

BfArM. (2023). *Digital health applications (DiGA)*. Federal Institute for Drugs and Medical Devices. https://www.bfarm.de/EN/Medical-devices/Tasks/Digital-Health-Applications/_node.html. Accessed March 15, 2025.

Brommeyer, M., Liang, Z., Whittaker, M., & Mackay, M. (2023). Developing health management competency for digital health transformation: Protocol for a qualitative study. *JMIR Research Protocols, 12*, e51884. https://doi.org/10.2196/51884

Butryn, T., Bryant, L., Marchionni, C., & Sholevar, F. (2017). The shortage of psychiatrists and other mental health providers: Causes, current state, and potential solutions. *International Journal of Academic Medicine, 3*(1), 5–9.

Car, J., Ong, Q. C., Erlikh Fox, T., et al. (2025). The digital health competencies in medical education framework: An international consensus statement based on a Delphi study. *JAMA Network Open*. https://doi.org/10.1001/jamanetworkopen.2024.53131

Ceballos-Espinoza, F. (2024). Reconstructive psychological assessment (RPA) applied to the analysis of digital behavioral residues in forensic contexts. *Journal of Criminal Psychology, 14*(4), 502–519. https://doi.org/10.1108/JCP-04-2024-0030

References

European Commission. (2022). *A European Health Data Space: Harnessing the power of health data for people, patients and innovation* (COM(2022) 196 final). Brussels. https://health.ec.europa.eu/system/files/2022-05/com_2022-196_en_0.pdf

Faria, M., Zin, S. T. P., Chestnov, R., Novak, A. M., Lev-Ari, S., & Snyder, M. (2023). Mental health for all: The case for investing in digital mental health to improve global outcomes, access, and innovation in low-resource settings. *Journal of Clinical Medicine, 12*(21), 6735. https://doi.org/10.3390/jcm12216735

Government of India. (2022). *National tele mental health programme*. Ministry of Health and Family Welfare.

Hajat, C., Hasan, A., Subel, S., & Noach, A. (2019). The impact of short-term incentives on physical activity in a UK behavioural incentives programme. *npj Digital Medicine, 2*, 91. https://doi.org/10.1038/s41746-019-0164-3

Holland Brown, T. M., & Bewick, M. (2022). Digital health education: The need for a digitally ready workforce. *Archives of Disease in Childhood. Education and Practice Edition.* https://doi.org/10.1136/archdischild-2021-322022

Hollis, C., Sampson, S., Simons, L., Davies, E. B., Churchill, R., Betton, V., Butler, D., Chapman, K., Easton, K., Gronlund, T. A., Kabir, T., Rawsthorne, M., Rye, E., & Tomlin, A. (2018). Identifying research priorities for digital technology in mental health care: results of the James Lind Alliance Priority Setting Partnership. *The Lancet Psychiatry, 8*(1), 41–50. https://doi.org/10.1016/S2215-0366(18)30296-7

Househ, M., Kushniruk, A. W., & Borycki, E. M. (Eds.). (2019). *Big data, big challenges: A healthcare perspective— Background, issues, solutions and research directions*. Springer. https://doi.org/10.1007/978-3-030-06109-8

Huang, Z., & Hu, Q. (2024). Tree hole rescue: An AI approach for suicide risk detection and online suicide intervention. *Health Information Science and Systems, 12*(1), 45. https://doi.org/10.1007/s13755-024-00298-3

Iorfino, F., Occhipinti, J. A., Skinner, A., Davenport, T., Rowe, S., Prodan, A., Sturgess, J., & Hickie, I. B. (2021). The impact of technology-enabled care coordination in a complex mental health system: A local system dynamics model. *Journal of Medical Internet Research, 23*(6), e25331. https://doi.org/10.2196/25331

Khaled, S. M., Al-Abdulla, M., Tulley, I., & others. (2024). Qatar's national mental health study—the World Mental Health Qatar. *International Journal of Methods in Psychiatric Research, 33*(S1), e2008. https://doi.org/10.1002/mpr.2008

Linardon, J., Fuller-Tyszkiewicz, M., Firth, J., et al. (2024). Systematic review and meta-analysis of adverse events in clinical trials of mental health apps. *Digital Medicine, 7*, 363. https://doi.org/10.1038/s41746-024-01388-y

Lui, G. Y., Loughnane, D., Polley, C., Jayarathna, T., & Breen, P. P. (2022). The apple watch for monitoring mental health-related physiological symptoms: Literature review. *JMIR Mental Health, 9*(9), e37354. https://doi.org/10.2196/37354

Malgaroli, M., Schultebraucks, K., Myrick, K. J., Loch, A. A., Ospina-Pinillos, L., Choudhury, T., Kotov, R., De Choudhury, M., & Torous, J. (2025). Large language models for the mental health community: Framework for translating code to care. *Lancet Digit Health, 7*, e283–e285. https://doi.org/10.1016/S2589-7500(24)00300-1

Martí Noguera, J. J. (2024). *Ethics in digital mental health*. Ethics Press. https://ethicspress.com/products/ethics-in-digital-mental-health

Mohr, D. C., Silverman, A. L., Youn, S. J., Areán, P., Bertagnolli, A., Carl, J., Carlton, T., Chaudhary, N., Cooper, D., DeVito, S., et al. (2025). Digital mental health treatment implementation playbook: Successful practices from implementation experiences in American healthcare organizations. *Front Digit Health., 7*, 1509387. https://doi.org/10.3389/fdgth.2025.1509387

NHS England. (2023). *Psychological therapies: Annual report on the use of IAPT services, England 2022–23*. NHS Digital.

Nordberg, S. S., Jaso-Yim, B. A., Sah, P., Schuler, K., Eyllon, M., Pennine, M., Hoyler, G. H., Barnes, J. B., Murillo, L. H., O'Dea, H., Orth, L., Rogers, E., Welch, G., Peloquin, G., & Youn, S. J. (2024). Evaluating the implementation and clinical effectiveness of an innovative digital first care model for behavioral health using the RE-AIM framework: Quantitative evaluation. *Journal of Medical Internet Research, 26*, e54528. https://doi.org/10.2196/54528

OECD. (2021). *A new benchmark for mental health systems: Tackling the social and economic costs of mental ill-health*. OECD Publishing.

OECD. (2024). *Futures of global AI governance: Co-creating an approach for transforming economies and societies*. OECD Publishing.

Pote, H., Rees, A., Holloway-Biddle, C., & Griffith, E. (2021). Workforce challenges in digital health implementation: How are clinical psychology training programmes developing digital competences? *Digital Health, 7*, 2055207620985396. https://doi.org/10.1177/2055207620985396

Pourat, N., Tieu, L., & Martinez, A. E. (2022). Measuring behavioral health integration in primary care. *Population Health Management, 25*(6), 721–728. https://doi.org/10.1089/pop.2022.0160

RAND Europe. (2022). The impact of vitality active rewards with apple watch on physical activity: Results from a longitudinal observational study of UK vitality members. Technical Report. https://www.vitality.co.uk/media/rand-2022-impact-vitality-active-rewards-apple-watch-physical-activity.pdf

Rony, M. K. K., Das, D. C., MostT, K., et al. (2025). Artificial intelligence in psychiatry: A systematic review and meta-analysis of diagnostic and therapeutic efficacy. *Digital Health, 11*. https://doi.org/10.1177/20552076251330528

Schmidt, L., Pawlitzki, M., Renard, B. Y., Klose, C., Frank, M., & Mühlhausen, M. (2023). The evolution of Germany's digital therapeutics reimbursement program. *Digital Medicine, 6*, 177. https://doi.org/10.1038/s41746-023-00837-4

Singapore Ministry of Health. (2023). *National mental health and wellbeing strategy*. MOH. https://isomer-user-content.by.gov.sg/3/15393410-a42b-45a8-af5f-e432e2e4342a/national-mental-health-and-well-being-strategy-report-2023.pdf

Sit, H. F., Chen, W., Wu, D., Huang, Y., Xu, D. R., & Hall, B. J. (2024). Digital mental health: A potential opportunity to improve health equity in China. Lancet. *Public Health, 9*(12), 10.1016/S2468-2667(24)00268-3.

Sit, N., Vernot, C., Littman, R., Voors, M., Meriggi, N. F., Abajobir, A., et al. (2023). COVID-19 and mental health in 8 low-and middle-income countries: A prospective cohort study. *PLoS Medicine, 20*(4), e1004081.

Tan, W. J., Larance, B., Schweickle, M. J., Lim, A. S. X., Lowe, K., & Kelly, P. J. (2025). Sociocultural context of SMART recovery in Singapore: A qualitative exploration of members and facilitators perspectives and experiences. *Drug and Alcohol Review*. https://doi.org/10.1111/dar.14048

Stroud, A. M., Anzabi, M. D., Wise, J. L., Barry, B. A., Malik, M. M., McGowan, M. L., & Sharp, R. R. (2025). Toward safe and ethical implementation of health care artificial intelligence: Insights from an academic medical center. *Mayo Clinic Proceedings: Digital Health, 3*(1), 100189. https://doi.org/10.1016/j.mcpdig.2024.100189

Titov, N., Dear, B. F., Staples, L. G., Bennett-Levy, J., Klein, B., Rapee, R. M., Andersson, G., Purtell, C., Bezuidenhout, G., & Nielssen, O. B. (2020). The first 30 months of the MindSpot Clinic: Evaluation of a national e-mental health service against project objectives. *Australian & New Zealand Journal of Psychiatry, 54*(7), 726–739. https://doi.org/10.1177/0004867419899979

Torous, J., Bucci, S., Bell, I. H., Kessing, L. V., Faurholt-Jepsen, M., Whelan, P., Carvalho, A. F., Keshavan, M., Linardon, J., & Firth, J. (2021). The growing field of digital psychiatry: Current evidence and the future of apps, social media, chatbots, and virtual reality. *World Psychiatry, 20*(3), 318–335. https://doi.org/10.1002/wps.20883

van Genderen, M. E., Kant, I. M. J., Tacchetti, C., & Jovinge, S. (2025). Moving toward implementation of responsible artificial intelligence in health care: The European TRAIN initiative. *JAMA*. https://doi.org/10.1001/jama.2025.1335

van Sonsbeek, M. A. M. S., Hutschemaekers, G. J. M., Veerman, J. W., Vermulst, A., & Tiemens, B. G. (2023). The results of clinician-focused implementation strategies on uptake and outcomes of Measurement-Based Care (MBC) in general mental health care. *BMC Health Services Research, 23*(1), 326. https://doi.org/10.1186/s12913-023-09343-5

Whitmyre, E. D., Esposito-Smythers, C., López, R., Jr., Goldberg, D. G., Liu, F., & Defayette, A. B. (2024). Implementation of measurement-based care in mental health service settings for youth: A systematic review. *Clinical Child and Family Psychology Review, 27*(4), 909–942. https://doi.org/10.1007/s10567-024-00498-z

World Health Organization. (2022). *World mental health report: Transforming mental health for all*. World Health Organization.

World Health Organization. (2023). Ethics and governance of artificial intelligence for health: Guidance on large multi-modal models. Geneva: WHO. https://www.who.int/publications/i/item/9789240074729

World Health Organization. (2024). *Psychological interventions implementation manual: Integrating evidence-based psychological interventions into existing services*. WHO. https://www.who.int/publications/i/item/9789240087149.

World Health Organization. (2025a). *Guidance on mental health policy and strategic action plans: Module 1. Introduction, purpose and use of the guidance*. WHO.

World Health Organization. (2025b). *Guidance on mental health policy and strategic action plans: Module 2. Key reform areas, directives, strategies, and actions for mental health policy and strategic action plans*. WHO.

World Innovation Summit for Health. (2024). WISH 2024: Humanizing Health: Conflict, Equity and Resilience. https://wish.org.qa/home/

Youn, S. J., Schuler, K., Sah, P., Jaso-Yim, B., Pennine, M., O'Dea, H., Eyllon, M., Barnes, J., Murillo, L., Orth, L., Hoyler, G., & Nordberg, S. (2025). Scaling out a digital-first behavioral health care model to primary care. *Administration and Policy in Mental Health and Mental Health Services Research*, 1–21. https://doi.org/10.1007/s10488-025-01433-2

Chapter 5
Governance and the Role of the Digital Behavioral Health Expert

5.1 Introduction: Bridging Governance and Implementation

This chapter examines the critical gap between governance frameworks and implementation practices in digital behavioral health. The successful implementation of digital technologies in mental healthcare requires a comprehensive governance model that guides AI use across the entire behavioral health ecosystem—a framework that the 5P Model (predictive, preventive, personalized, participatory, and precision-based care) potentially offers under human oversight. While previous chapters have established the theoretical foundations of the 5P Model, this chapter focuses on the practical challenges of translating these principles into operational reality and introduces how human expertise becomes essential to bridge this governance-implementation gap.

The Implementation Gap in Digital Behavioral Health
The 5P Model provides a comprehensive governance framework, but even the most well-designed governance structures fail without effective implementation. As Cabitza et al. (2020) demonstrate in their analysis of AI implementation in healthcare, technically sophisticated systems frequently fail to deliver value when faced with what they term the "last mile" implementation gap. This gap manifests in two fundamental challenges:

1. **The Hiatus of Human Trust**: When frontline providers and patients distrust digital interventions or perceive them as secondary to traditional care, implementation fails regardless of the system's technical capabilities. Mohr et al. (2025) document this phenomenon extensively in their digital mental health implementation playbook, noting that "the fragility of trust among referring

providers" can rapidly erode when clinicians perceive digital tools as threats rather than extensions of their practice. Their research reveals that "one or two negative comments from patients can quickly undermine confidence" in digital interventions.
2. **The Hiatus of Machine Experience**: The quality of digital systems depends entirely on the quality of data that informs them. As Cabitza notes, "No algorithm, no matter how smart or intelligent it is, can produce value if its input lacks value in the first place." Mohr's implementation research identifies "data integration" as a critical challenge, noting that while "full integration of digital mental health data into the EHR allows for seamless data sharing," this integration is often delayed by practical constraints.

These implementation gaps are particularly challenging in digital behavioral health because they occur at the intersection of clinical, technical, and governance domains. Traditional mental health professionals were trained for a fundamentally different paradigm—one where knowledge was centralized in clinical expertise rather than distributed across technical systems, where governance was primarily institutional rather than algorithmic, and where interventions were episodic rather than continuous.

Value-Driven Implementation Frameworks

Bridging the governance-implementation gap requires more than technical deployment—it demands a fundamental reconsideration of how value is defined and measured. As Bohler et al. (2024) demonstrate, conventional value-based care models risk becoming "a wolf in sheep's clothing" when they fail to account for social determinants, potentially exacerbate disparities, and increase administrative burdens without corresponding benefits.

Effective implementation of the 5P Model requires establishing value frameworks across multiple dimensions:

- **Clinical Value**: Implementing predictive and precision systems that demonstrably improve outcomes through quantifiable metrics (e.g., reduced wait times, improved symptom scores, decreased rehospitalization)
- **Operational Value**: Implementing preventive workflows that enhance efficiency and coordination, reducing administrative burden while improving care continuity
- **Economic Value**: Implementing participation models that demonstrate cost-effectiveness through prevention of high-acuity interventions and more efficient resource utilization

Mohr's implementation research confirms the importance of defining explicit "key performance indicators" across these dimensions, with "clearly defined goals and targets" that guide implementation efforts.

5.1 Introduction: Bridging Governance and Implementation

Data Governance as Implementation Infrastructure
Data governance serves as the essential infrastructure for implementing the 5P Model. Drawing from Cabitza et al.'s framework, effective implementation requires addressing six key data governance challenges:

1. **Standardization and Consensus**: Implementing standardized data protocols that maintain governance intent across clinical settings while preserving necessary clinical flexibility
2. **Inter-rater Reliability**: Developing governance practices that address variations in clinical documentation and interpretation, ensuring sufficient consistency for reliable algorithm performance
3. **Data Work Support**: Designing processes that support the essential human work of data generation and validation, recognizing it as core clinical activity rather than administrative burden
4. **Human-Computer Interface Design**: Ensuring that digital interfaces enhance rather than impede clinical workflows, supporting the usability needs identified by Mohr et al. as critical to implementation success
5. **Data Management**: Establishing secure and accessible data repositories that enable the predictive and personalized elements of the 5P Model
6. **Strategic Data Governance**: Guiding continuous improvement of data quality and utilization, aligning with the participatory component of the 5P Model

These data governance activities transform abstract governance principles into concrete implementation infrastructures.

Implementation Mechanisms for the 5P Model
Bridging governance principles and implementation practices requires clear, replicable mechanisms. While Mohr et al.'s implementation framework offers a pragmatic lens, it should be contextualized within broader digital mental health governance imperatives. The following five mechanisms reinterpret and expand on Mohr's categories in alignment with the 5P Model:

1. **Value Translation and Performance Alignment**
   Implementation begins with a shared understanding of success. In the 5P framework, key performance indicators (KPIs) are not merely metrics—they are governance anchors that link predictive capacity with public value. Drawing from Nilsen et al. (2023) and WHO's Module 5 (2025a), KPIs should reflect health equity, usability, and participatory outcomes, not just clinical throughput.
2. **Multilevel Stakeholder Synchronization**
   Effective implementation demands "governance readiness" across systems. This includes aligning national strategies, clinical workflows, and digital infrastructure—a principle rooted in adaptive governance and supported by cross-sector

frameworks (Auf et al., 2025; WHO, 2025b). Engagement is reframed as capability building—not just buy-in but capacity sharing.

3. **Data Standards as Governance Instruments**
   Quality protocols are not only technical specifications—they are mechanisms of trust. In the 5P Model, data quality ensures predictive reliability and ethical personalization. This includes interoperable data infrastructures (Nordberg et al., 2024) and contextualized standards for AI accountability (Microsoft Research, 2024; EU AI Act, 2024).
4. **Adaptive Governance and Learning Cycles**
   Rather than static rollout plans, 5P implementation relies on continuous learning systems. These mirror learning health system logics, where predictive insights feed preventive interventions in real time (Friedman et al., 2017). Adaptation becomes a governance function—not just operational refinement.
5. **Governance-Driven Feedback Loops**
   Feedback in 5P systems is multidirectional. Patients, providers, and platforms contribute to iterative change. This requires both technical tools (e.g., dashboards, decision support) and sociotechnical structures (e.g., participatory review boards, DBHE-led ethical audits). It aligns with Mohr's emphasis on champions but extends toward *collective governance literacy*.

Phased Implementation Strategy for the 5P Model

Implementation is not linear—it unfolds through cycles of *learning, adaptation, and system integration*. A phased strategy allows each 5P pillar to be activated contextually:

1. **Pilot Phase: Codesign and Cultural Readiness**
   Rather than solely testing tool efficacy, early pilots should assess governance capacity: ethical oversight mechanisms, DBHE coordination, and readiness indicators for platform integration (WHO, 2024). Mohr's insights on "innovation-minded champions" can be reframed as early adopters of *governance-aligned innovation*.
2. **Scaling Phase: Institutional Integration and Interoperability**
   Scaling requires not just technical deployment but *cross-actor alignment*—including funders, regulators, and platform providers. This phase benefits from lessons in regional digital therapeutic expansion (e.g., DiGA, Tele-MANAS, PBH models) which have demonstrated the importance of *interoperability across care layers* (Nordberg et al., 2024; Auf et al., 2025).
3. **Sustainability Phase: Embedding Ethical Feedback and Decommissioning Logic**
   Sustainability involves more than maintenance. It includes the authority to *decommission ineffective tools* (a governance function), redistribute resources, and refine value-aligned indicators. This is a key insight from equity-centered frameworks (Robinson et al., 2024) and implementation science (Nair et al., 2024).

This phased approach recognizes that implementing the 5P Model is not a linear technical deployment but an iterative process requiring continuous governance adaptation.

The Workforce Challenge
The implementation challenges identified in this chapter point to a critical workforce gap: the absence of professionals specifically equipped to bridge clinical, technical, and governance domains in digital behavioral health. While existing professionals remain essential to mental healthcare delivery, they were not trained to navigate the dimensional complexity of implementing the 5P Model.

The following sections will explore how a new professional role—specifically designed to bridge governance and implementation—could address the challenges identified in this chapter, providing a strategic workforce solution for operationalizing the 5P Model in digital behavioral health.

5.2 Capacity Building for Sustainable 5P Implementation

The operational success of the 5P Model depends not only on deploying the right technologies but on building the human, ethical, and systemic capacity to govern those technologies wisely, equitably, and sustainably. Implementation, in this sense, is not a purely technical endeavor—it is a process of building the institutional maturity, professional roles, and cultural legitimacy needed to support new forms of care.

While global frameworks such as DECODE and WHO's digital health competencies offer shared reference points, their application must remain flexible and responsive to local realities. Behavioral health systems are shaped by diverse historical, social, and cultural dynamics. As such, capacity building must integrate both generalist competencies—such as ethical oversight, digital literacy, and systems thinking—and context-specific knowledge, including sociocultural values, community governance practices, and regional priorities in mental health.

This section introduces five interdependent building blocks for sustainable implementation:

- Professional competencies (Sect. 5.2.1)
- Value governance (Sect. 5.2.2)
- Ethical oversight of AI (Sect. 5.2.3)
- Systemic integration (Sect. 5.2.4)
- Governance readiness: from mental health to behavioral ecosystems (Sect. 5.2.5)

Together, they offer a flexible but structured roadmap for activating the 5P Model in real-world behavioral health ecosystems—across sectors, disciplines, and cultural contexts.

Transition Note: From Governance Theory to Implementation Practice As outlined in Chap. 4, the Digital Behavioral Health Expert (DBHE) is not a traditional clinician or technician—it is a strategic governance role designed to embed, align, and sustain the 5P Model across digital behavioral health ecosystems. This section now marks the shift from theory to practice: from understanding why the DBHE is needed to exploring how the role can be developed, implemented, and scaled. Section 5.2.1 introduces the DBHE's core competencies and system functions, forming the foundation for readiness assessment tools (Sect. 5.2.5), system integration strategies (Sect. 5.2.4), and institutional pathways for sustainable scaling (Sect. 5.3.3).

5.2.1 Human Infrastructure: The DBHE Role and Core Competencies

The Digital Behavioral Health Expert (DBHE) represents a new kind of professional scaffolding—not a replacement for existing roles but a structural response to the evolving demands of behavioral health in a digitally mediated environment. As systems shift from episodic, clinician-centered care to continuous, AI-augmented, and data-driven models, existing professionals face a widening gap between their training and the operational realities of digital behavioral health.

This transformation creates three overlapping workforce needs:

- Reskilling: Helping traditional professionals navigate and engage with digital workflows, governance models, and platforms
- AI Literacy: Cultivating the ability to understand, interrogate, and collaborate with algorithmic systems
- Upskilling: Developing advanced competencies in governance, cross-sector translation, and the cocreation of ethical, value-aligned digital ecosystems

As Nair et al. (2024) highlight, a critical gap persists in our understanding of the actual responsibilities and activities of leaders during the AI implementation process. This leadership vacuum is not merely operational—it reflects the absence of well-defined, accountable roles capable of navigating the intersections of clinical, ethical, and technological domains. The study underscores the urgent need for new professional functions trained to steward AI systems across the full implementation life cycle, from design to monitoring and adaptation. In this light, the DBHE role is not a theoretical construct but a necessary response to the systemic fragmentation of responsibilities in digital mental health governance.

The DBHE stands at the intersection of these needs. It is not merely a new technical role—it is a translation infrastructure that enables ethical, effective, and scalable implementation of the 5P Model across health systems. In this sense, the DBHE operates as a human integrator: facilitating alignment between technology and clinical goals, between patient experience and platform design, and between governance structures and innovation pathways.

Critically, the emergence of the DBHE reflects a broader shift in how behavioral health is conceptualized:

- From care as an individual encounter to care as a continuous, data-supported process
- From professionals as primary knowledge holders to distributed intelligence across humans and systems
- From static roles to fluid, interdisciplinary capacities that evolve alongside technologies and ethical expectations

In addition, the DBHE role is inherently AI collaborative, designed not only to operate alongside large language models (LLMs) and other AI-driven agents but to actively govern and coevolve with them. This professional does not merely supervise automated systems—they function as augmented actors within a constellation of intelligent agents, many of which are capable of generating content, triaging requests, and adapting over time. The DBHE becomes a co-orchestrator of hybrid agency, continuously aligning machine learning systems with clinical ethics, user dignity, cultural relevance, and policy frameworks. This is not a role designed to replace human expertise but to ensure that AI becomes a tool for care, not a source of friction or displacement. Like *R2D2* in the *Star Wars* universe—a quiet but essential system actor who coordinates, alerts, and safeguards operations—the AI agents in digital behavioral health systems are embedded, not leading. The DBHE ensures they serve, not displace, human priorities.[1]

The DBHE also differs fundamentally from other roles in that it is AI-native trained. Like air traffic controllers, DBHE professionals are selected and trained not simply based on qualifications but on task-specific capacities that are not universally trainable. The complexity, situational awareness, and ethical demands of the role require individuals with exceptional coordination and abstraction abilities and who can integrate technical fluency with clinical and governance knowledge. Importantly, the DBHE operates under continuous monitoring and reflective supervision to ensure quality, accountability, and iterative learning.

Training a DBHE is therefore not a commodity-based or time-based educational process. It is a *value-based investment*, where the cost of training is directly related to the impact generated through more effective implementation, reduced risk, and accelerated system integration. As with aviation, the investment in training reflects the *strategic importance and risk profile* of the environment being governed.

---

[1] *R2D2* is a fictional character from the *Star Wars* film series, widely recognized as a non-humanoid AI agent that assists human actors by managing critical systems and navigation tasks. The metaphor is used to illustrate how AI agents in digital health can act in assistive roles without replacing human agency or decision-making.

This evolution demands a new competency architecture. To ensure legitimacy and transferability, DBHE competencies are mapped onto two validated frameworks:

1. The European DECODE Framework for digital competence (especially in information literacy, safety, collaboration, and digital problem-solving)
2. The ethical governance framework from *Ethics in Digital Mental Health* (Martí-Noguera, 2024), emphasizing trust, transparency, equity, and human dignity in tech-mediated care (Table 5.1)

Table 5.1 Core competencies of the DBHE aligned with the 5P Model

5P dimension	DBHE core competency	Metaphor or example	What it enables
Predictive	AI literacy and governance	Like a food safety inspector, the DBHE does not design the algorithm but ensures it is safe, fair, and understandable	Ensures ethical and effective use of AI tools for early detection and risk stratification
Preventive	Value governance	Like a conductor who ensures harmony without playing every instrument, the DBHE coordinates actors around shared goals	Aligns diverse stakeholders to define what matters before problems escalate—enabling preventive design
Personalized	Digital systems navigation	Like an urban planner retrofitting smart roads into old cities, the DBHE integrates tools into existing workflows	Makes digital tools usable, relevant, and adapted to individual care pathways
Participatory	Cross-sector mediation	Like a multilingual interpreter in a high-stakes negotiation, the DBHE bridges clinicians, developers, and managers	Fosters collaboration, cocreation, and human-centered implementation
Precision	Equity and cultural competence	Like a local guide in a diverse ecosystem, the DBHE adapts systems to different realities, identities, and communities	Increases adoption, trust, and accuracy by contextualizing digital interventions

> **The DBHE as Airspace Controller: A Systemic Role for 5P Governance**
> To understand the function of the Digital Behavioral Health Expert (DBHE), imagine the digital behavioral health ecosystem as a complex airspace. In this airspace, clinicians, AI systems, mental health platforms, patients, and policymakers are all "pilots" navigating different missions—delivering care, processing data, generating insights, or ensuring regulation. The DBHE acts as the air traffic controller, maintaining real-time coordination and governance of this shared environment. See an example in Table 5.2.

(continued)

5.2 Capacity Building for Sustainable 5P Implementation

Table 5.2 An example for DBHE acting as the air traffic controller

5P Model	Airspace metaphor	DBHE contribution
Predictive	Predictive analytics = radar detection of incoming issues	Anticipates risks by overseeing AI and early-warning systems
Preventive	Coordinated flight paths prevent collisions	Aligns tools and workflows to reduce errors, duplication, or gaps in care
Personalized	Each plane has a unique route and destination	Ensures tools are adapted to patient needs and integrated into individualized pathways
Participatory	Pilots, towers, and ground staff coordinate continuously	Facilitates communication between clinicians, patients, IT teams, and administrators
Precision	Aircraft operate under precise altitudes, speeds, and times	Ensures data, decisions, and digital actions are timely, relevant, and context specific

Crucially, the DBHE does not replace existing roles—just as an air traffic controller does not fly the planes or engineer the aircraft. Instead, the DBHE enables other professionals to operate more safely, collaboratively, and effectively within a complex digital health environment. By managing this "behavioral health airspace," the DBHE enhances the impact of:

- Clinicians, by reducing digital friction and surfacing relevant insights
- Technologists, by translating ethical and clinical needs into actionable requirements
- Patients, by supporting trust, usability, and rights in digital systems
- Managers and policymakers, by aligning operational and governance priorities

The DBHE provides the coordinating intelligence and ethical navigation needed to make the 5P Model operational—not as an external force but as part of an integrated care and governance team.

Just as air traffic controllers operate not in 2D maps but in four-dimensional airspace, the DBHE governs in a digital environment where platforms move in space and time, where ethical decisions depend on predictive futures, and where human dignity is protected in real time and asynchronously.

5.2.2 Value Governance as a New Implementation Skill

Most implementation frameworks focus on tools, workflows, or training. Few address the core question: what are we implementing, and why does it matter? In the 5P Model, implementation is not a neutral process—it is a form of value orchestration. That orchestration requires a skillset: value governance.

Value governance refers to the intentional processes by which digital systems are aligned with shared definitions of value. It is not just about outcome measurement—it is about who defines success, whose needs are centered, and how decisions are sustained over time and across platforms.

In digitally mediated behavioral health, value governance must be:

- **Multidimensional**: spanning clinical, ethical, operational, human, and strategic value
- **Participatory**: co-defined with stakeholders, not imposed from above
- **Dynamic**: capable of adapting to new evidence, technologies, and risks

Without this framing, digital systems default to technical throughput and invisible bias. AI systems may optimize for engagement but not for dignity. Interventions may increase efficiency but widen inequity. The DBHE is trained to detect, prevent, and realign these tendencies.

This concern is echoed by international efforts to rethink governance models. Mental health systems are increasingly shaped by algorithmic logic, and yet most remain unequipped to embed governance capacity beyond compliance. The World Economic Forum's (2021, 2022) toolkits similarly stress the need to build trust "into" digital systems, not around them—yet they stop short of defining the professional roles that would make such trust operational.

Reframing Value for Managers and Investors

While value governance benefits patients and providers, its greatest under-leveraged benefit may be for those financing, managing, or scaling health systems.

The economic justification for value governance is compelling. Recent critiques of value-based healthcare payment models (Bohler et al., 2024) highlight how simplistic value metrics can become "a wolf in sheep's clothing" when they hold providers accountable for outcomes determined largely by social factors beyond their control. These critiques resonate because they expose a fundamental misalignment: value is being defined too narrowly, with inadequate attention to implementation contexts.

This misalignment creates direct financial consequences:

- Implementation failure rates reach 70% in digital health initiatives (Damschroder et al., 2009; Mohr et al., 2025).
- Workforce burnout increases when clinicians are held to metrics they cannot influence, accelerating costly turnover.
- Disengagement from digital tools wastes substantial technology investments.
- Avoidance of complex patients drives unintended costs elsewhere in the system.

For managers and investors, value governance represents a protective strategy against these losses. By establishing multidimensional value from the outset—not just clinical outcomes but operational efficiency, strategic differentiation, and

5.2 Capacity Building for Sustainable 5P Implementation

reduced regulatory risk—organizations create the conditions for sustainable returns on digital investments.

Unlike traditional ROI frameworks that position value as a distant, uncertain outcome, value governance tracks and manages value creation from implementation day one. It ensures that:

- Capital expenditures align with organizational mission
- Clinical and technical teams share outcome goals
- User adoption is designed in, not hoped for
- Risk is managed continuously, not reactively
- Systems generate value across multiple timescales—from immediate operational benefits to long-term strategic positioning

Value governance accelerates not just time to value but also time to trust—an increasingly scarce currency in digital mental health. Crucially, it creates the foundation for ethical revenue growth—particularly important in mental health, where trust directly impacts utilization and retention. Organizations with robust value governance report higher patient loyalty, clinician retention, and sustained competitive advantage in digital transformation.

Operationalizing Value: A New Role in Health System Logic
In traditional models, value was defined externally (by funders or administrators), assessed late (at the end of interventions), and often reduced to cost-effectiveness or clinical throughput. In the 5P Model, value is defined early, with patients, communities, and system actors, and continuously governed throughout the life cycle of the intervention.

The DBHE plays three essential functions in this space:

- **Value Translator**: connecting diverse actors—patients, AI teams, clinicians, policymakers—around a shared language of value
- **Value Steward**: ensuring that ethical, human, and community values are not lost during scaling, automation, or optimization
- **Value Integrator**: aligning predictive systems, data flows, and decision-making tools with evolving definitions of meaningful impact

Example
In a system deploying AI-based triage, value governance means asking: "Are we optimizing for speed or for equity? For clinical urgency or community needs? Who decides what constitutes a risk worth flagging?"

Yet value governance faces a paradoxical barrier: naming it creates resistance, while digital systems advance by default. Most digital transformations do not begin with stakeholder consensus—they happen quietly, through design choices, interface defaults, and system adoption. Platforms become indispensable before their implications are fully debated.

By contrast, when governance is named—when roles like the DBHE are introduced or when systems pause to define value collectively—resistance often follows. Not because the governance is incorrect but because making value visible interrupts the seamless flow of tech adoption. It demands critical attention where most digital systems thrive on frictionless use.

The DBHE is trained not to provoke dialogue for its own sake but to govern attention, shape defaults, and channel behavioral patterns toward ethically aligned and value-coherent outcomes. Their function is not to manage controversy but to preconfigure choice architectures that embed equity, transparency, and user dignity into the system itself.

This paradox can be summarized as follows:

> **Frictionless Systems, Invisible Power**
> - Digital tools succeed not because they are better but because they are easier.
> - Governance begins when you name what technology renders invisible: purpose, risk, exclusion, values.
> - The DBHE is not there to slow things down but to ensure what moves fast does so in the right direction.

The Value Governance Cycle
To make value governance operational, the DBHE implements a continuous cycle with four key components:

1. **Value Definition**: Engaging diverse stakeholders to establish what constitutes value across all five dimensions in specific contexts
2. **Value Architecture**: Designing technical, procedural, and organizational structures that embody and protect defined values
3. **Value Measurement**: Creating metrics that make value visible across dimensions, going beyond clinical or economic measures
4. **Value Adaptation**: Establishing processes for continuous learning and adjustment as technologies and contexts evolve

This cycle provides a structured framework for what otherwise might remain abstract—ensuring that value is not just articulated but actively governed throughout implementation.

Navigating Dimensional Value
Like the black hole metaphor that opens this chapter, value exists in a warped dimensional space where what appears simple on the surface conceals complex gravitational forces below. The DBHE functions as a navigator of this dimensional complexity—sensing the forces that pull behavior, data, and decision-making in particular directions and recalibrating the system to maintain ethical alignment.

5.2 Capacity Building for Sustainable 5P Implementation

The value governance cycle translates this philosophy into a structured process—clarifying not only what value means but how it is activated and maintained over time. Through this continuous process of definition, architecture, measurement, and adaptation, value becomes not just an aspiration but an operational reality that evolves with the system.

In systems governed by throughput and scale, value is often assumed—rarely interrogated. The DBHE disrupts this pattern by embedding governance into design, making space not for ideological contestation but for deliberate alignment. At this stage of digital development, the architecture has already been built—what remains is to humanize the walls. As life designers of the behavioral health ecosystem, DBHE professionals ensure that digital structures are not just operational but meaningful. In the next section, we examine how this same DBHE-led orientation applies to one of the most volatile areas of digital transformation: the ethical oversight of AI.

Global Governance Guidance: What Is Missing?
International frameworks increasingly emphasize the importance of ethics in digital mental health:

- OECD (2024) calls for governance models that go beyond compliance, noting that mental health systems must be equipped to manage algorithmic risks and build equity by design.
- World Economic Forum (2021, 2022) promotes "trust architecture" and shared standards for digital mental health, advocating transparency, explainability, and stakeholder inclusion.

However, despite their value, these frameworks remain largely conceptual. They outline *what* ethical digital systems should achieve but not *who* implements, monitors, or governs them. The role of the Digital Behavioral Health Expert (DBHE) addresses this critical gap, offering the human infrastructure necessary to translate global governance principles into operational practice.

Rather than duplicating existing standards, the DBHE enables systems to *inhabit them*—bridging policy, practice, and people across evolving digital ecosystems.

5.2.3 *From Ethical Oversight to Cultural Stewardship: Health Ethics in a Digital Age*

While Chap. 4 illustrated the systemic need for embedded ethics through real-world implementation cases, this section explores how ethical oversight becomes an operational capacity within the DBHE role. Ethics here is not reactive—it is a strategic, relational, and cultural function that must be sustained over time and across systems.

Ethics has become a central word in the global digital health conversation—frequently invoked yet inconsistently defined. In the context of digital behavioral health, ethics is not merely a set of abstract principles; it is a set of operational decisions made in environments marked by uncertainty, power asymmetries, and evolving technologies. AI ethics must move beyond abstract declarations and become embedded in the design and operation of digital health systems, particularly in environments of low transparency and high asymmetry. This operational perspective becomes increasingly critical as algorithms begin to mediate access to care, triage decisions, and even therapeutic content, elevating the stakes of ethical governance exponentially.

At the same time, digital systems introduce new risks: algorithmic bias, opaque decision-making, unintended exclusion, and surveillance creep. Ethical failures in these domains do not just harm individuals—they erode trust in entire systems. As the WHO (2021) warns, "Ethical lapses in AI systems can lead to systemic trust collapse, with implications far beyond technical malfunction, particularly in public health ecosystems." In response, the Digital Behavioral Health Expert (DBHE) acts as a sentinel—not to block innovation but to channel it in ways that reinforce fairness, transparency, and human dignity.

In this ethically complex landscape, the role of DBHE does not serve as an abstract guardian of universal principles. Rather, the DBHE is a human actor, embedded in their time and cultural context, who operates with awareness of both possibility and constraint. Their role is not to substitute care with compliance nor to eliminate uncertainty but to build systems where digital mediation reinforces, rather than undermines, human dignity and institutional trust.

This requires three crucial recognitions:

- **Ethical oversight is not omniscient.** No framework can anticipate all risks. The DBHE must work iteratively, learn from failure, remain transparent about trade-offs, and foreground the lived experiences of affected communities.
- **The goal is not perfection—it is alignment.** Ethical governance is about reducing the gap between system behavior and human intention. That gap can never fully close, but it can be narrowed through thoughtful design, participatory feedback, and systemic humility.
- **Collaboration trumps control.** The DBHE is not a solo actor imposing rules on others. Instead, they co-govern with developers, clinicians, patients, and managers—prompting collective inquiry, guiding deliberation, and translating ethical priorities into operational decisions. As UNESCO (2021) affirms, "Ethical governance must be participatory and pluralistic, engaging diverse societal actors including patients, communities, and professionals in co-decision processes."

This is not a technical task—it is a cultural one. The DBHE is not expected to code systems but to prompt, guide, and contextualize the work of those who do. Their fluency lies in the ethical dimensions of digital design, not the syntax of programming languages.

> **Ethical Governance Is Not a Firewall**
> - Ethics is not a boundary to keep technology out—it is an *architecture* that defines how technology participates in care.
> - The DBHE does not delay innovation—they *redirect it* toward inclusion, accountability, and sustainable trust.
> - Ethical oversight is not neutral—it always reflects a position. The DBHE makes that position *explicit, debatable, and improvable*.

They are not replacing human care—they are governing the conditions under which digital systems enter, shape, or exit the care process.

The idea that ethics must "participate from within" aligns with UNESCO's framing of ethics as embedded infrastructure—not a constraint but a condition for legitimate and trustworthy innovation. As Auf et al. (2025) underscore in their scoping review of AI use in mental health decision-making, ethical participation must be embedded early and iteratively in system design to avoid replicating institutional blind spots or excluding vulnerable groups from algorithmic logic.

The DBHE as Cultural Transition Agent

As demonstrated in Chap. 4, digital behavioral health systems are not merely adding tools—they are undergoing a *paradigm shift*. Governance is no longer contained within professional silos or fixed workflows; it now emerges at the intersection of AI behavior, platform dynamics, regulatory uncertainty, and lived experience. In this transitional space, the DBHE becomes a *cultural integrator*—not enforcing universal rules but holding space for ethical reflection, negotiation, and alignment. As the WHO (2023) emphasizes, "Cultural adaptation and ethical reflection must be integral to the governance of AI in health to avoid reinforcing colonial or technocratic logics."

The DBHE supports health systems in:

- Moving from *reaction to anticipation*
- Evolving from *procedural ethics to reflexive governance*
- Shifting from *control-oriented leadership to sensemaking and stewardship*

In short, the DBHE does not represent a new layer of compliance but a new kind of professional intelligence—one that makes *ethical meaning operational* across diverse and distributed digital environments.

> **Ethics Is Not Universal: Navigating Cultural Perspectives in a Digitally Mediated World**
> In a globally interconnected mental health ecosystem, ethics is not a one-size-fits-all model—it is a *relational practice* grounded in values, social histories, institutional trust, and cultural norms. Digital systems may operate across borders, but what is considered ethical still depends on where and how people live, heal, and relate to systems of care.

Table 5.3 Examples of cultural variation in ethical dimensions of digital mental health systems (Adapted from UNESCO, 2021)

Ethical dimension	Example of cultural variation
Autonomy	In some care systems, individual choice is central; in others, family or community-based decision-making is prioritized
Privacy	While some frameworks emphasize data ownership and consent, others focus on relational transparency and trust management
Harm	In some regions, algorithmic bias raises concerns; in others, exclusion due to language, infrastructure, or stigma is more salient
Trust	Nudging technologies may be seen as helpful guidance in some settings and as undue influence or surveillance in others
Governance legitimacy	The authority to define what is "ethical" may rest with regulatory bodies, community leaders, health professionals, or even technology developers—depending on institutional history and public engagement

UNESCO (2021) recognizes that ethics must be guided by local norms and cultural diversity. This includes autonomy, privacy, harm, trust, and legitimacy as context-dependent categories. These dimensions are interpreted differently across care systems, institutional traditions, and sociotechnical environments, as illustrated in Table 5.3.

As emphasized by UNESCO (2021), ethics must be shaped through local norms, social histories, and lived experiences—not universal abstractions. Ethical pluralism is not a threat to consistency but a prerequisite for legitimacy.

- The DBHE is not tasked with enforcing one ethical framework but with *mediating across perspectives*, recognizing cultural tensions, and building shared understanding through situated governance practices.

Ethical governance, in this light, is not an *imported checklist*—it is a *co-constructed system of alignment* that evolves with context. For this reason, the DBHE must be equipped not only with digital and clinical fluency but also with intercultural competence, reflexivity, and governance empathy.

Opening Ethical Governance to Collective Dialogue

This section, and the broader governance framework it contributes to, does not aim to close ethical debates with definitive conclusions. On the contrary, it represents an invitation: to question, critique, and reimagine what ethical oversight means across geographies, disciplines, and lived experiences.

We have deliberately refrained from offering a formalized reference canon, as the current landscape of globally cited frameworks remains dominated by Euro-American institutions. Rather than reinforce that imbalance, we invite further work to surface, center, and integrate governance knowledge rooted in African, Asian, Indigenous, and community-based traditions. This book does not present the final word—it offers an open call to codevelop a plural, situated, and adaptive ethics of digital mental health.

5.2.4 System Integration: Driving Value in a Fragmented Landscape

In digital behavioral health, systemic integration is often described as a technical problem—interoperability, platform connectivity, and secure data sharing. But at its core, integration is a value problem. It requires systems to be coherent not only in infrastructure but in purpose. As established in Chap. 1, tech companies now function as governance actors across infrastructure, algorithm, and interface layers. This multilayered governance ecosystem demands a role specifically designed to ensure alignment between these layers—the DBHE.

System Integration Pain Points: Why Fragmentation Persists

Despite significant investment in digital mental health, systemic integration faces persistent barriers that transcend any single technology or implementation:

1. **Lack of Global Vision**: Organizations typically optimize for departmental or episodic outcomes rather than system-wide transformation. Each stakeholder sees only their part of the elephant—IT focusing on security, clinicians on workflow, and administrators on cost. Without a role designed to maintain the global vision, implementations fragment into competing priorities.
2. **Siloed Interests and Incentives**: Different actors in the behavioral health ecosystem operate with fundamentally misaligned incentives. Platform companies prioritize user retention and engagement metrics, clinicians value therapeutic alliance and evidence-based practice, while funders focus on cost containment and measurable outcomes. These competing interests create governance friction that technology alone cannot resolve.

3. **Shortage of Cross-Domain Expertise**: Most professionals are trained within a single domain—clinical, technical, or managerial. Few possess the interdisciplinary fluency to translate across these domains, interpret their distinct value frameworks, and align their divergent priorities. This expertise gap becomes particularly acute when implementing technologies that operate across traditional boundaries.
4. **Misalignment in Investment Governance**: Both public and private funding mechanisms tend to finance discrete digital "solutions" rather than integrated governance capacity. Without investment in roles that orchestrate alignment between tools, equity considerations, and sustainable implementation, even well-funded innovations remain isolated and short-lived.

Integration Approaches: Global Implementation Examples
Different healthcare systems have developed varied approaches to addressing these integration challenges, each with distinctive strengths and limitations:

Singapore's Integration Model As discussed in Chap. 4, Singapore's Smart Nation mental health initiative exemplifies strong alignment across predictive, preventive, personalized, and precision-based dimensions of the 5P Model. Their approach centralizes data governance while distributing implementation through local health clusters. A key innovation has been the establishment of cross-functional teams that include clinical informaticians, AI ethicists, and implementation specialists who function in DBHE-like roles. As noted in Chap. 1, Singapore's use of AI-powered early detection systems demonstrates how predictive tools can be integrated into population health infrastructure, though participatory governance remains an area for continued development (Singapore MOH, 2023).

Saudi Arabia's National Strategy Referenced in Chap. 4, the Saudi approach demonstrates strong integration between predictive, preventive, and participatory elements. Their national mental health transformation program has innovated by creating regional integration hubs where digital systems are adapted to local cultural and religious contexts through formal codesign with community leaders, clinicians, and technical teams. As highlighted in Chap. 2, this approach represents a distinctive economic model that balances central investment with localized implementation, though gaps remain in personalization and precision-based implementation (Almubarak & Alhabeeb, 2024).

Australia's Dimensional Coordination Australia's approach, examined in Chap. 4, demonstrates sophisticated integration of predictive and preventive elements through Iorfino et al.'s (2021) system modeling research. As discussed in Chap. 3, their work aligns with sociotechnical systems theory by showing how digital platforms can enable early intervention and care coordination that outperforms both traditional and telehealth models. However, their implementation reveals integra-

5.2 Capacity Building for Sustainable 5P Implementation

tion gaps in personalization, participation, and precision—highlighting the challenge of moving from research models to fully operationalized systems.

These examples illustrate a critical pattern: even well-designed national strategies struggle to achieve comprehensive integration across all five dimensions of the 5P Model. The gaps are not random but reflect systemic governance challenges that require new professional capacities to address.

The economic transformation articulated in Chap. 2 highlighted how digital economics have evolved from pay-once models to continuous-service economies. This shift creates a critical governance challenge: how to ensure that value flows to all stakeholders in these continuous service models, not just platform owners. The DBHE addresses this by ensuring that economic incentives align with clinical and ethical requirements, preventing the risk of value extraction without corresponding benefit to patients and communities.

Where most roles optimize parts of the system—a product, a pathway, a protocol—the DBHE operates across domains. They are not a replacement for IT architects, clinicians, or health managers. But they are the only actor designed to understand and align the logic of all three and to ensure that the invisible forces driving digital adoption—algorithmic priorities, stakeholder incentives, engagement metrics—do not derail ethical, clinical, or cultural alignment.

Case Comparisons: Where 5P Integration Succeeds and Fails

A review of international implementations highlights the variability in how different systems interpret and operationalize the 5P Model. Table 5.4 offers a high-level comparative snapshot of selected national strategies and pilot programs, mapping their alignment with each of the five governance components.

Table 5.4 Global alignment with the 5P governance model: a comparative snapshot

Country/case	P1: Predictive	P2: Preventive	P3: Personalized	P4: Participatory	P5: Precision based
Australia/Iorfino et al.	✓	✓	☐	☐	☐
Germany/DiGA	☐	☐	✓	☐	✓
India – Tele-MANAS	✓	✓	☐	✓	☐
Singapore – Early Detection	✓	✓	✓	☐	✓
Saudi Arabia – Nat. Strategy	✓	✓	☐	✓	☐
China – Tree Hole Rescue	✓	✓	☐	☐	✓
USA/Youn et al.	✓	✓	✓	✓	✓
WHO/Guidance 2025a–e	☐	✓	☐	✓	☐

✓ = Strong alignment | ☐ = Partial or potential alignment

Note on Methodology and Interpretation This comparative table is the result of a structured but non-exhaustive review of current literature, strategic plans, and selected implementation studies as referenced throughout Chaps. 1–4. It is intended to illustrate patterns of alignment with the 5P governance model—not to offer a definitive or evaluative ranking. Gaps or partial alignments may reflect evolving programs, limited public documentation, or shifting policy focus. Any inaccuracies are unintentional and should be viewed as an invitation for further dialogue and refinement by local experts and system stakeholders.

Questions for Readers and Systems Thinkers
- Why do most national strategies invest heavily in predictive and preventive tools but neglect participatory or personalized components?
- What are the political, infrastructural, or cultural barriers to systemic *upskilling*—particularly in roles like the DBHE that transcend traditional boundaries?
- How can integration be governed if each component (P1–P5) remains in a different silo?
- Where are the opportunities to embed a role that orchestrates alignment, ensures ethical coherence, and maximizes value across this matrix?

This comparative analysis reveals a critical pattern: even well-funded and technically sophisticated national initiatives rarely achieve strong alignment across all five dimensions of the 5P Model. The gaps are not random but reflect systemic challenges in governance. Without a role specifically designed to bridge these gaps, implementation remains fragmented—strong in some areas but underperforming in others.

What does true integration require?

- Domain coordination: linking digital, clinical, and policy workflows
- Incentive alignment: clarifying why each actor participates and for what return
- Temporal phasing: sequencing changes to avoid disruption and enabling learning
- Governance embedment: ensuring that ethics, oversight, and quality assurance are built-in—not retrofitted

The DBHE is not solely responsible for these shifts. But they are the only role whose competencies explicitly prepare them to see the full integration map and guide it with governance intelligence.

Digital mental health systems often focus on services: triage bots, screening tools, e-therapy apps. But the DBHE is trained to focus on systems: the flow of data across jurisdictions, the alignment of tools with governance and patient rights, and the structural readiness of institutions to evolve over time. This directly addresses the polycentric governance challenge identified in Chap. 3, where multiple centers of decision-making operate with varying degrees of autonomy.

They help answer questions that bridge the theoretical frameworks of Chap. 3 with the practical implementation challenges of Chap. 4:

- How do predictive tools work across cultural or policy boundaries?
- Are ethical frameworks operational or just aspirational?

5.2 Capacity Building for Sustainable 5P Implementation

- Can systems scale without sacrificing personalization or safety?

This is not abstract. It is investment logic. The comparative analysis above shows that even well-designed 5P implementations can fail when they lack the integration capacity to sustain governance across all five dimensions. Integration without governance leads to failure, duplication, risk, and waste. Investing in integration means investing in the roles that make it possible.

> **Governance Integration Questions for Investors and Policymakers**
> - Are we building digital systems that scale safely across populations and geographies?
> - Who ensures that ethical frameworks evolve with tools and do not remain static?
> - Can implementation adapt to changing regulatory or cultural environments?
> - Are we investing in roles that align the value chain or just the tech chain?

When we examine the cases in Table 5.1 through the lens of system integration, we see that only the US implementation (Youn et al., 2025) achieved strong alignment across all five dimensions—and this was in a controlled implementation with substantial resources and cross-disciplinary leadership. This pattern confirms that comprehensive 5P governance does not happen by chance—it happens through deliberate cultivation of roles like the DBHE that can operate in the dimensional space described at the beginning of this chapter.

Without a DBHE or equivalent role, integration depends on goodwill and coincidence. With the DBHE, integration becomes strategic, measurable, and ethically sound. As we navigate the increasingly complex airspace of behavioral health data and digital systems, the DBHE becomes not just beneficial but essential—the coordinating intelligence that ensures safe navigation across dimensions, domains, and disciplines.

Taken together, the elements outlined in this section—human infrastructure, value governance, ethical oversight, and systemic integration—do not merely constitute building blocks for implementation. They represent the emergence of a new capability paradigm in behavioral health governance: one that is anticipatory, adaptive, and deeply aligned with the multidimensional nature of care in the digital age. The DBHE is not a patch for existing gaps; it is a strategic actor designed for a world where technology, ethics, population needs, and governance imperatives converge in real time. As systems move from experimentation to scale, the question is no longer whether we need such roles but how we develop, deploy, and sustain them. The next section turns to this challenge, exploring what it means to *scale what works*, not only in technology but in human capacity to govern it well.

5.2.5 Governance Readiness: From Mental Health to Behavioral Ecosystems

While Sect. 5.2.4 focused on system integration across existing healthcare domains, this section addresses a more fundamental transition that digital transformation necessitates. The preceding sections established how the DBHE navigates cross-domain complexity and supports integration within current healthcare structures. However, as we now explore, there is a deeper shift underway: the expansion of governance beyond traditional mental health into the broader realm of behavioral ecosystems.

As governments worldwide invest in mental health infrastructure, most policies, budgets, and frameworks continue to define the challenge narrowly—focusing on mental health as a clinical or diagnostic issue. Yet digital platforms, AI systems, and behavior-based interventions increasingly govern much more than mental illness. What is at stake is the governance of behavioral health: a broader, data-intensive domain encompassing emotions, cognition, social patterns, and digital traces.

This distinction is critical. Behavioral health captures what people do, not just how they feel or how they are diagnosed. As such, it touches everything from digital interactions and workplace behavior to sleep patterns, family dynamics, and platform engagement. And as digital tools increasingly mediate these dimensions, institutions must ask: Governance of what? If we continue designing governance systems for "mental health" alone, we will miss the broader sociotechnical shift that is already underway.

To better understand this conceptual shift, Table 5.5 contrasts traditional mental health governance with the emerging behavioral health governance paradigm. This comparison highlights the expanded scope, actors, and approaches required when governing behavioral ecosystems rather than just clinical mental health services.

Table 5.5 Mental health vs. behavioral health governance readiness

Dimension	Mental health governance	Behavioral health governance
Focus	Diagnoses, therapy, clinical treatment	Emotional, cognitive, social, and digital behaviors
Scope	Psychiatry, psychology, care delivery	Schools, tech platforms, families, public health
Primary actors	Clinicians, insurers, medical regulators	Developers, community leaders, educators, patients
Data source	Symptoms, clinical notes, diagnostic codes	Passive sensing, app usage, wearables, social signals
Risks	Misdiagnosis, stigma, access gaps	Algorithmic exclusion, surveillance creep, overreach
Governance tools	Ethics committees, guidelines, legal frameworks	Algorithm audits, participatory design, digital accountability mechanisms
Role of DBHE	Absent or ad hoc	Central to bridging gaps and ensuring ethical coherence

> **Governing What?**
> - Most national strategies still speak the language of mental health governance.
> - But AI, platforms, and behavioral nudges now operate beyond clinical boundaries.
> - Behavioral governance involves new domains, new actors, and new risks.
> - It demands a distinct readiness logic—not just in funding but in how institutions think.

This table makes clear: governing behavioral health is not an extension of clinical governance—it is a different problem space. It requires new tools, broader coalitions, and institutional imagination.

The DBHE plays a critical role in enabling this shift. They help organizations evolve from a compliance-based logic focused on mental illness to an adaptive logic focused on behavioral complexity. This means:

- Translating existing protocols into multi-context systems
- Mapping ethical risks that do not appear in clinical settings
- Building readiness across technical, social, and cultural axes

To systematically assess an organization's ability to govern in this expanded behavioral ecosystem, we need a structured approach to governance readiness evaluation. The following framework provides both diagnostic and developmental guidance for systems transitioning to behavioral health governance.

Why Governance Readiness Matters

Across national contexts, health systems often deploy digital tools with the assumption that access to technology equates to transformation. However, Chap. 4's case studies repeatedly illustrate that the impact of digital systems depends not on their technical features but on the governance capacity surrounding them.

Governance readiness refers to a system's institutional ability to absorb, adapt, and scale ethically governed digital care models. It is not a binary state but a spectrum—varying across structural, cultural, and procedural dimensions. Understanding this readiness is essential to avoid premature scale-up, wasted investments, and ethical backlash.

Four Dimensions of Governance Maturity

To structure this analysis, we propose four interdependent dimensions of governance maturity. Together, they form a diagnostic tool for system capability and a roadmap for investment in workforce and institutional transformation.

- **Structural Capacity**
  - Are there designated entities or funded mechanisms responsible for digital behavioral health governance?
  - Are roles like the DBHE structurally embedded in teams, programs, or policies?
- **Process Maturity**
  - Are there defined and iterative processes for ethical review, feedback integration, and oversight adaptation?
  - Can governance evolve in response to context-specific risks?
- **Cultural Legitimacy**
  - Does the governance system hold trust among professionals, users, and communities?
  - Are local values, languages, and social norms reflected in design and decision-making?
- **Collaborative Intelligence**
  - Can actors across clinical, technical, regulatory, and civil society sectors coordinate effectively?
  - Are there shared vocabularies, data structures, and implementation workflows?

Building on these four dimensions, Table 5.6 presents a maturity model for behavioral health governance systems. This developmental framework helps organizations assess their current state and identify targeted investments needed to advance their governance capabilities.

Table 5.6 Stages of governance maturity in digital behavioral health systems

Maturity stage	System description	Role of the DBHE	Typical system characteristics
Initial	Governance is reactive, siloed, or informal	Absent or ad hoc	Low trust, tech-led logic, fragmented oversight
Emerging	Basic advisory functions in place	External consultant or pilot role	Partial coordination, early-stage ethics protocols
Operational	Oversight is institutionalized	Embedded DBHE in delivery teams	Ethical governance, shared metrics, adaptive review
Strategic	Governance shapes innovation	DBHE leads implementation strategy	Cross-sectoral alignment, real-time feedback loops
Embedded	Governance is identity defining	DBHE in leadership and system design	Transnational integration, system reflexivity, cultural legitimacy

Note: This framework reflects a developmental continuum. A system may be advanced in one domain (e.g., structural capacity) but nascent in others (e.g., cultural legitimacy). Governance maturity must be evaluated holistically and iteratively

DBHE Readiness Assessment: Practical Application Tool

To operationalize the governance maturity model presented in Table 5.7, organizations need practical tools for self-assessment. The following diagnostic framework provides a simplified entry point for evaluating DBHE implementation readiness:

Interpretation

- **4–6**: Early stage readiness—Focus on awareness building and foundational governance structures.
- **7–9**: Intermediate readiness—Consider pilot implementation with external DBHE consultation.
- **10–12**: Advanced readiness—Proceed with full DBHE implementation with internal capacity development.

This simplified assessment serves as an initial diagnostic, with comprehensive evaluation methodologies available through further engagement. By identifying their current position on this readiness spectrum, organizations can more strategically invest in the capability development needed to maximize returns on digital transformation initiatives.

From Readiness to Return: Why Investment in Maturity Pays Off

Investing in governance maturity is not a compliance cost—it is a strategic enabler of system transformation. High-readiness systems demonstrate:

- Lower failure rates in implementation
- Faster time to value for digital investments
- Higher stakeholder engagement and institutional trust
- Greater adaptability to cultural, regulatory, and technological change

Table 5.7 DBHE implementation quick assessment matrix

Dimension	Basic (1)	Developing (2)	Advanced (3)	Score
Structural integration	No formal digital governance mechanisms	Digital oversight exists but operates in silos	Cross-functional governance structures with clear accountability	
Digital literacy	Limited awareness of AI risks and capabilities	Some technical understanding but gaps in governance implications	Comprehensive understanding of both technical and ethical dimensions	
Value alignment	Focus on technical implementation only	Recognition of multiple value streams but not integrated	Structured approach to balancing clinical, human, ethical, and strategic value	
Cross-domain coordination	Siloed operations between clinical and technical teams	Basic coordination mechanisms but frequent friction	Systematic translation and collaboration across domains	

As outlined in Sect. 5.2.4, many global implementations stall not because tools are poorly designed but because governance capacity is underdeveloped. This is a risk management problem: without readiness, digital systems drift toward.

> **Readiness Is Not Readiness to Buy but Readiness to Govern**
> - Governance maturity is not defined by tool acquisition or IT budgets.
> - True readiness is the capacity to align digital capabilities with public interest and human dignity.
> - The DBHE does not manage procurement but builds the scaffolding that allows systems to evolve responsibly.

This expanded governance scope represents a critical evolution beyond what previous sections have addressed. While Sect. 5.2.1 established the DBHE's core competencies, Sect. 5.2.2 explored value governance as an implementation skill, Sect. 5.2.3 examined ethical oversight in digital environments, and Sect. 5.2.4 focused on system integration across healthcare domains, none of these fully captured the *conceptual expansion* of what we are governing. The governance readiness framework presented here does not simply repeat these earlier discussions of integration and implementation—it fundamentally reframes their scope and application.

The importance of this distinction becomes clear when considering how the DBHE role operates in practice. A DBHE focused only on integrating traditional mental health services with digital tools would miss critical governance opportunities in behavioral ecosystems: school-based emotion recognition systems, workplace wellness platforms, or social media mental health nudges. These hybrid spaces—neither purely clinical nor purely technological—represent the frontier where governance innovation is most urgently needed.

In closing, governance readiness is no longer just about capacity—it is about clarity. Systems must be ready not only to govern digital health but to understand what is being governed. Without this clarity, investment in digital tools may outpace the ethical and institutional ability to use them responsibly. The DBHE ensures that this readiness is not aspirational but operational, trainable, and scalable.

Having examined the five foundational capacities for 5P Model implementation—professional competencies, value governance, ethical oversight, system integration, and governance readiness—we now ask: How can these capacities be institutionalized across entire systems, not just pilots?

Section 5.3 focuses on sustainable, system-wide transformation. It outlines how the DBHE role and 5P logic can be embedded within governance infrastructures, enabling long-term alignment between ethics, innovation, and public value across this expanded behavioral ecosystem.

5.3 Beyond Implementation: Building a Global Standard for Digital Behavioral Health Governance

This final section shifts from reflection to proposition. The previous chapters outlined why current governance frameworks fall short, what capacities are needed to overcome these limits, and how the DBHE role can be embedded into systems that are increasingly mediated by AI and platforms. But a question remains—one that any serious policymaker, educator, or institutional leader will ask after reading this book:

How Do We Get This Profile?
The previous sections (Sects. 5.2.1–5.2.5) outlined the core capacities needed to make 5P implementation possible: new professional roles (DBHE), value governance, embedded ethics, cross-system integration, and governance maturity. But capacity alone is not enough. Transformation happens when those capacities become part of institutional logic—woven into workforce planning, platform design, and national policy. That is the purpose of this section.

Yet the institutional context is shifting. As Chap. 1 established, behavioral health is no longer governed solely by ministries, hospitals, or clinical authorities. Instead, much of its architecture—data storage, risk scoring, access pathways, behavioral nudges—is now designed and controlled by digital platforms, AI systems, and engagement infrastructures that operate outside the public sector. This is not just a new toolset. It is a reconfiguration of governance itself.

The pace of digital transformation often outstrips institutional reflexes. While behavioral health systems slowly adapt their policies and roles, platforms advance silently—embedding engagement architectures, refining algorithmic triage, and defining what counts as a mental health need. By the time public institutions recognize this shift, many key governance decisions have already been made—by others, in code, and at scale.

The 5P Model and the DBHE role respond to this reality. They are not designed for pilot projects or siloed programs. They are designed to be embedded—modular, adaptable, and aligned with national and cross-sectoral strategies for governing behavioral health in the age of AI.

At the core of this transformation is a difficult truth: governments are racing to deploy AI in healthcare, but many do so without the capacity to govern what they are adopting—let alone what they no longer own. Public institutions are attempting to manage data-driven behavioral ecosystems using frameworks built for episodic, professionally mediated care.

If transformation is to be sustainable, it must happen at the level of infrastructure, not just implementation. Institutionalizing the 5P Model means embedding governance logic directly into the algorithms, workflows, and platform layers where behavioral health is now mediated. It means preparing systems not only to use AI but to guide, adapt, and align it with public interest.

We are living through an infrastructural shift where governance no longer belongs exclusively to professions or institutions—it is becoming borderless. Platforms govern behaviors across nations. AI systems scale interventions without geographical boundaries. In this new landscape, the governance logic must be equally scalable—adaptable across cultures, sectors, and regulatory frameworks yet consistent in protecting human dignity.

This is the function of a *Global Public Behavioral Health School*—not as a physical campus but as a transnational coordination mechanism. Its mission: Define a standard for DBHE training that is culturally adaptable, ethically grounded, and operationally precise.

A Global Standard for the DBHE Role
Why does this matter?

Because no single country, company, or clinician can govern behavioral health in isolation anymore.

- Behavioral signals flow across borders.
- AI models trained in one region are deployed in another.
- Governance failures in one platform affect trust across the ecosystem.

A global DBHE standard ensures:

- Consistency in ethical and technical competencies
- Cultural adaptability for diverse populations and norms
- Scalability of 5P governance logic across systems
- Alignment between local action and global responsibility

Why Standards Must Emerge Now
The urgency is clear. AI is not waiting for slow institutional deliberation. From LLM-powered triage bots to emotion-sensing wearables, the tools are already here. What is missing is trained human intelligence embedded in the loop—people with the legitimacy, capacity, and vocabulary to govern these tools in context.

Standards Are Not Bureaucracy. They Are Infrastructure.
- A standard defines what must be upheld—even when systems change.
- Without standards, governance depends on personal ethics, not institutional design.
- A DBHE standard protects patients, systems, and technologies from silent drift (Table 5.8).

Table 5.8 Five domains a global DBHE standard should cover

Domain	Why it matters
Governance intelligence	Ability to operate in hybrid systems, across legal, clinical, and platform boundaries
Ethical fluency	Competence in situational ethics, AI risk, equity frameworks, and community-centered values
AI collaboration	Skills to evaluate, translate, and govern machine learning models and interfaces
System integration	Capacity to connect workflows, stakeholders, and data environments across silos
Cultural mediation	Reflexivity to adapt interventions and oversight to local norms and lived realities

A Modular Vision, Not a Monopoly
This proposal does not require a new WHO department or a single university's monopoly. Instead, it proposes a distributed, modular model—a set of reference competencies, adaptable training pathways, and shared governance principles that any country, platform, or health system can adopt and localize.

Like Creative Commons or ISO certifications, this model enables coherence without demanding conformity.

A Final Word to the Reader
If you are a policymaker, this book invites you to invest not just in technology but in the human intelligence to govern it well.

If you are a clinician, this book invites you to recognize governance as care and the DBHE as your partner.

If you are an investor or platform designer, this book invites you to align innovation with trust—by embedding ethics where your system decisions are made.

And if you are someone—like the author—without institutional power, working at your kitchen table, this book was written with you in mind. Because digital behavioral health will shape lives everywhere, and its governance must include the wisdom, courage, and clarity of those often left out.

From 5P to Shared Power
In behavioral health, the future is not just digital—it is relational. The DBHE is not a controller of systems but a connector of worlds. The 5P Model is not a framework of prediction but of participation. And the transformation we offer here is not a disruption—it is a new form of care.

Governance is not a side task. It is the work of deciding what we value, how we act, and who gets to shape the systems we all live in.

Section 5.3.1 engages directly with the institutional realities of AI integration in behavioral health. Section 5.3.2 frames governance not as ownership but as alignment in systems we do not control. Sections 5.3.3–5.3.4 build the transition logic from role to standard to institutional design.

5.3.1 Strategic Foundations: Why a Global Standard

The institutional reality of behavioral health is no longer defined by hospitals, ministries, or clinical authorities alone. Much of its architecture—data storage, triage algorithms, engagement infrastructures—is now shaped by digital platforms, often governed outside the traditional public sector. In this landscape, governance can no longer be limited to professional licensing or institutional oversight. It must become infrastructural, embedded, and adaptive.

This is why the 5P Model and the Digital Behavioral Health Expert (DBHE) role must be translated into a global standard. Not as a bureaucratic requirement but as a *governance logic*—modular, ethical, and culturally adaptive. The question is no longer whether this is needed but *how* to build it in a way that aligns global coherence with local legitimacy.

Digital behavioral health is already governed but not always visibly, not always accountably, and, increasingly, not by public actors. As AI systems guide triage, platforms mediate emotional expression, and data infrastructures preconfigure eligibility for care, governance no longer operates from within the clinic or state. It now unfolds through architectures, protocols, and predictive systems that often lie beyond the reach of national policy. This section reframes the notion of a "global standard" not as a regulatory imposition nor a Western export but as a strategic coordination scaffold: a way to surface shared thresholds, clarify distributed responsibilities, and sustain value-based alignment in a health ecosystem increasingly shaped by digital actors.

Governance Without Ownership

The most urgent governance challenge in digital behavioral health is not the absence of regulation—it is the misalignment between systems. Clinical AI systems developed in one country are deployed in another, often without adjustment. Platforms designed to optimize engagement are repurposed for emotional support or behavioral nudging. Meanwhile, global institutions like WHO, OHCHR, and UNESCO—once central to setting public health ethics—are now repositioning themselves as facilitators of AI innovation under the pressures of scalability and crisis (Strange & Tucker, 2024). This governance vacuum is not just institutional—it is infrastructural. It creates an asymmetry in which ethical intentions remain locally articulated, while system behaviors are globally distributed and unaccountable.

From Ethical Drift to Strategic Anchoring

The proliferation of AI-enabled systems in mental healthcare has introduced new forms of ethical drift. Fairness is declared but not audited. Bias is acknowledged but not mitigated. Consent becomes a checkbox, not a process. As Näher et al. (2023) warn in their analysis of secondary health data systems, these inconsistencies deepen inequity, especially for underserved populations already absent from dominant data infrastructures. The risk is not that AI or data-driven systems fail but that they succeed without shared commitments to equity, trust, and participation. In such environments, governance must shift from compliance to anchoring: from late-stage review to embedded alignment with purpose.

5.3 Beyond Implementation: Building a Global Standard for Digital Behavioral Health...

This shift has already begun to materialize in frameworks like the Artificial Intelligence–Quality Implementation Framework (AI-QIF), which reframes implementation not as a technical rollout but as a value-aligned process codesigned with stakeholders to ensure contextual legitimacy and ethical fidelity across systems (Nilsen et al., 2023).

A global standard for the Digital Behavioral Health Expert (DBHE) role, and the competencies that support it, offers such an anchor. But it cannot be a static framework. It must function as a situated infrastructure for coordination—adaptable across contexts, interoperable across systems, and legitimate across sectors. Its purpose is not to control what others build but to ensure that value governance, ethical reflexivity, and cultural adaptability remain present wherever behavioral health is digitized.

Four Strategic Shifts for Coherent Governance

These four shifts are not abstract theory—they are strategic orientations already emerging in diverse systems, from India to the United States and from public policy to private innovation:

1. **From Ad Hoc to Anticipatory**
   Most digital behavioral health tools are deployed reactively: pilot first, governance later. The first strategic shift is to embed anticipatory thresholds into systems from the outset. The DBHE standard provides modular evaluation tools to assess whether a digital mental health intervention aligns with all five dimensions of the 5P Model: predictive, preventive, personalized, participatory, and precision based. Such anticipatory logic is central to the design of the AI-QIF, which begins its implementation journey with systemic reflection and cocreation, embedding foresight into each of its 14 steps before deployment even begins (Nilsen et al., 2023).

2. **From Compliance to Competency**
   Ethical guidelines are not enough if the systems implementing them lack the human capacity to interpret, adapt, and operationalize them. The standard defines the competencies required for this translation. These are not abstract ethical ideals—they are situated practices that connect predictive logic with clinical reasoning, technical functionality with lived experience, and system goals with user dignity. This emphasis on lived, actionable competency is echoed in frameworks that seek to define the operational capacity required for ethical AI deployment in healthcare—notably, in the AI-QIF, which identifies both the relational and technical skills needed for successful, context-sensitive implementation (Nilsen et al., 2023; Nair et al., 2024).

3. **From Ownership to Stewardship**
   AI governance is often framed in terms of data ownership. But ownership does not equal power nor does it ensure alignment. In digital behavioral health, where platform actors often operate outside traditional clinical systems, governance requires a shift from control to *stewardship*. Consent architectures, audit trails, metadata equity, and *federated learning (FL)* are emerging as key infrastructures of trust (Arefin et al., 2025).

> **Federated Learning as Stewardship Infrastructure**
> Federated learning (FL) is a privacy-preserving infrastructure already piloted in mobile health, mental health apps, and cross-institutional AI collaborations. Rather than centralizing sensitive behavioral health data, FL enables each organization to train models locally and share only anonymized updates. These are then aggregated into a shared model that improves accuracy and equity—without compromising patient privacy or data sovereignty.
>
> This approach has been used to:
>
> - Enhance personalization in *mental health mobile apps*
> - Enable *telehealth platforms* to collaborate without sharing raw video or session data
> - Support *cross-border AI development* without violating data protection laws like GDPR
> - Improve *digital phenotyping* tools while keeping users' behavioral traces private
>
> In behavioral health, FL is more than a technical fix. It represents *embedded governance*—a distributed, plural, and scalable way to align AI development with ethical, legal, and cultural priorities.

Federated learning is a decentralized approach to machine learning that allows organizations to collaborate on AI model development without sharing raw data. Instead of pooling sensitive behavioral health data into a central repository, each institution trains the model locally and only shares anonymized updates. These updates are then aggregated to improve a shared model—enhancing accuracy and equity while protecting privacy and data sovereignty.

This approach is particularly well-suited to behavioral health systems, where ethical concerns, regulatory constraints, and cultural diversity make centralized data strategies risky and often inappropriate. FL offers not just a technical solution but a governance redesign: it aligns with principles of local autonomy, plural knowledge, and distributed control.

Seen through this lens, federated learning becomes a *paradigm of stewardship*. It shows how coherence and collaboration can be achieved *without ownership*. As described in *Ethics in Digital Mental Health* (Martí-Noguera, 2024), FL allows clinics in different regions or countries to codevelop predictive models while maintaining local control over their data. This decentralization enhances both *trust and equity*, especially in systems vulnerable to surveillance, bias, or exclusion.

In this model, governance does not follow design—it *is* the design. It is not enforced through compliance alone but *cocreated through infrastructural choices*—guided by values, competencies, and localized knowledge. FL demonstrates how *modular, aligned standards*, implemented by DBHE-trained professionals, can enable ethical, scalable, and culturally adaptive governance in a borderless digital ecosystem.

4. **From Institutional to Infrastructural**
   Institutions alone can no longer govern the behavioral health ecosystem. App developers, data processors, wearable manufacturers, and AI-as-a-service providers now shape the architecture of care but are rarely held to health-specific governance standards. A global DBHE standard must recognize these actors not as adjacent stakeholders but as co-constructors of behavioral health systems. This means developing interoperable protocols, joint accountability mechanisms, and shared ethical thresholds that operate across clinical and nonclinical domains. This distributed approach to governance mirrors the strategic insights gathered in cross-national studies on AI implementation, which highlight the urgent need for flexible, context-aware standards that can operate beyond institutional silos (Nair et al., 2024).

   Governance, in this model, is not about inviting new players to existing forums—it is about redefining the forum itself, embedding ethical, participatory alignment within the architectures that drive care, engagement, and eligibility.

A Value-Based Standard, Not a Universal Rule

The DBHE standard is not a finished model to be transferred from center to periphery. It is a distributed diagnostic tool, a flexible scaffold, and a value proposition. It enables governments, platforms, and communities to ask the same foundational questions in different ways:

- What counts as value here?
- Who is accountable for it?
- How do we govern across systems we do not fully own?

This is not governance by control. It is governance by capability.

The standard emerges not from consensus but from alignment across difference. Its power lies not in uniformity but in creating the conditions for multiple actors—governments, technologists, clinicians, communities—to recognize each other across the asymmetries of the digital ecosystem.

This is how the DBHE role becomes operational—not as a new profession waiting for accreditation but as an already-emergent function asking to be resourced, protected, and scaled.

To translate the DBHE role into a scalable global reality, we must begin not with enforcement but with shared understanding. A global standard cannot emerge from templates or transfer—it must be cultivated through a common language: for competencies, for governance alignment, and for ethical implementation. In this sense, the proposed Global Public Behavioral Health School is not a peripheral training body—it is the first infrastructural step toward value-aligned, culturally adaptive governance.

In an age where digital infrastructure shapes emotional, cognitive, and relational life, governance can no longer be an afterthought. It must be the design. And shared standards are where that design begins.

5.3.2 Toward a Common Language: The School as First Step

Standards require shared understanding. To translate the DBHE role into a scalable global reality, we need a *common language*: for competencies, for governance alignment, and for implementation across diverse systems. The proposed *Global Public Behavioral Health School* is not merely a training institution—it is a first infrastructural step toward global coordination. It will define, validate, and adapt the DBHE standard—ensuring it is both culturally grounded and operationally precise.

> Why a Global Public School? To set a global standard for the DBHE? Yes—but also to correct a deeper imbalance. AI in behavioral health is shaping the future while therapists are overburdened and structurally excluded from digital governance. Are we just enriching AI while leaving professionals behind? It depends on healthcare economics. The School trains a new professional profile to accompany profiles like digital care navigators (DCNs), ensuring that this famous "human oversight" becomes real.

But the answer is not only to train new professionals. The School also enables current ones—therapists, regulators, policymakers—to reenter the conversation. It provides a structured response to a fragmented landscape where AI advances faster than institutional readiness. In doing so, it does not replace jurisdictional strategies—it helps align them.

This educational imperative is grounded in systemic realities: both well-resourced and underserved systems face misalignments between clinical training and digital implementation. While some systems struggle with sheer workforce scarcity, others face burnout, role confusion, and a lack of digital readiness. Professionals are trained for face-to-face episodic care, while digital systems now function as what could be called "meta-companions"—extending beyond clinical sessions to provide continuous monitoring, support, and early intervention. This gap between professional training and technological reality creates the exact governance void the School aims to address through interdisciplinary collaboration among "mental health professionals, engineers, lawyers, and economists" who together can establish the ethical foundations for responsible AI integration.

In an increasingly fragmented regulatory landscape, building a global standard for digital behavioral health governance requires more than technical convergence—it demands a shared language. A language not just of clinical excellence or AI safety but of value, equity, and institutional coherence. The proposed *Global Public Behavioral Health School* is the first step in creating that language.

This is not just a school. It is a *governance infrastructure*—a public, distributed, and adaptive mechanism to align global ambitions with local realities. It will define, validate, and evolve the *DBHE standard*, building on emerging cross-jurisdictional efforts like those documented by Chakraborty and Karhade (2024). Their comparative legal analysis of 14 AI governance frameworks—including those from Brazil, India, Singapore, China, Rwanda, and the EU—shows increasing alignment around the WHO's ethical principles: transparency, documentation, risk management, intended use, data quality, and privacy. Yet alignment does not mean harmonization.

From Jurisdiction to Coordination

The current patchwork of national strategies—including sector-agnostic laws, binding regulations, and guidance documents—reveals a shared momentum but fragmented implementation. There is no consensus on the definition of AI, let alone on how to validate clinical AI or operationalize risk thresholds across contexts. Definitions vary (e.g., Japan frames AI as abstract and context bound), and legal provisions diverge, even when citing the same WHO principles. Harmonization, then, must be a *cocreated process,* not a top-down export.

This is precisely where the *School* enters: not as an arbiter of norms but as a *platform for interoperability.* It enables health ministries, technologists, clinicians, and communities to align around modular standards, contextual validation methods, and culturally attuned implementation models. Through training, case-based learning, and codevelopment labs, it transforms regulatory insight into practical governance capability.

The Empathy Imperative: Beyond Algorithmic Intelligence

Empirical evidence reinforces the urgency of this infrastructure. A groundbreaking study by Jaso-Yim et al. (2024) demonstrated that digital care navigators (DCNs) increased registration rates for digital mental health interventions from 61.9% to 76.9%, with the most dramatic success (96.8% registration) occurring when human contact happened on the same day as referral. This "human touch" factor was not just about technical support—most conversations focused on building trust and comfort with digital systems.

Yet DCNs primarily address technical adoption, not governance. This points to a deeper need articulated by Gill (2024): the fundamental distinction between cognitive empathy (which AI can simulate) and emotional empathy (which motivates authentic care). AI systems can recognize patterns and respond according to protocols but cannot experience the emotional resonance necessary for genuine concern—creating what Montemayor et al. (2022) warn could become "psychopathic machines."

The School addresses this limitation by training DBHEs who bridge the cognitive-emotional gap. As Jeffrey (2016) notes, effective healthcare requires "an iterative process of emotional resonance and curiosity about the meaning of a clinical situation for the patient." This cannot be algorithmically simulated—it must be cultivated as a professional practice.

Toward Evidence-Aligned Standards

The School will curate and adapt evidence from global regulatory analyses—like Chakraborty and Karhade's comparative work—to inform:

- **Culturally grounded risk management** (e.g., Rwanda's focus on local data readiness; Japan's concept of "data economic zones")
- **Transparent clinical validation frameworks** (e.g., Singapore's metrics for PPV and LR−; India's adoption of CONSORT-AI and SPIRIT-AI)
- **Distributed privacy and accountability mechanisms** (e.g., federated learning as a design pattern for stewardship)
- **Empathy-based governance models** that acknowledge the fundamental limits of AI in emotional understanding while maximizing human-AI collaboration

These are not theoretical ideals. They are *jurisdictional experiments* already underway, ready to be synthesized into a living standard—codeveloped with and for those who govern, use, and build digital behavioral health systems.

Standards as Shared Capability

In line with the 5P governance model, the School supports a *capability-based approach to governance*, not a rule-based one. It trains DBHEs to serve as ethical anchors across systems they may not own, in infrastructures they may not have built, yet whose behaviors they are accountable for guiding.

Digital care navigators (DCNs) already exemplify this shift. As shown in recent implementation studies (e.g., Jaso-Yim et al., 2024), DCNs drastically improve engagement and access in digital systems—not by replacing technology but by making it human. Registration rates increase by up to 96.8% when navigators reach out the same day; drop-off is steep if delayed beyond 5 days. DCNs mitigate digital

5.3 Beyond Implementation: Building a Global Standard for Digital Behavioral Health...

illiteracy, bridge workflows, and humanize access. Yet they remain adjuncts to a clinical model unsuited for AI-driven ecosystems.

The DBHE complements them—not from above, but beside—embedding governance where it is most fragile: at the junction of data, design, and decision-making. It is through the partnership between DCNs and DBHEs that the 5P principles—predictive, preventive, personalized, participatory, and precision based—become not just rhetoric but operational infrastructure.

As recent frameworks warn (e.g., Malgaroli et al., 2025; Martí-Noguera, 2024; WHO, 2023; UNESCO, 2021), LLM deployment without governance-literate professionals risks not only clinical misfires but structural exclusion. Platforms scale, but human safeguards do not—unless governance is embedded through roles like the DBHE.

To ensure real human oversight, we must govern both the AI and the institutions around it. And that means training not just DCNs or DBHEs but creating an ecosystem that supports them both. Systems and people, working together, can drive smarter and more equitable investments in behavioral health. That is the role of the School: a blueprint for structural readiness, not just curriculum.

The tension between professional detachment and emotional connection described by Gill (2024) is particularly relevant here. Health professionals often face an expectation that being "professional" requires detachment, yet patients need their providers to express authentic care. The DBHE training addresses this tension directly, equipping professionals to maintain appropriate boundaries while ensuring systems remain human-centered. Like the "reciprocal experience" of empathy described in clinical settings, governance must be a reciprocal process—responsive to both technological capabilities and human needs.

In a world where AI regulation ranges from proactive (EU) to permissive (Singapore) to top-down (China), the School fosters *interoperability without uniformity*. It supports jurisdictions in adapting shared governance logics—like those aligned with WHO, OECD, and ITU guidance—into context-specific operational strategies.

The School is a public good. It supports not only workforce development but also policy innovation, multistakeholder dialogue, and alignment across regulatory, clinical, and technical domains.

In short, the School is not a theoretical exercise—it is the institutional counterpart to the very gaps this chapter has mapped. It operationalizes the call for readiness, capability, and ethical infrastructure introduced in Sects. 5.2.1–5.2.5. And it answers the question we posed at the beginning of this chapter: *how do we ensure this transformation benefits the many, not the few?*

5.3.3 Implementation Pathways: From Concept to Operational Reality

The Global Public Behavioral Health School represents a foundational step toward translating the DBHE role from conceptual framework to operational reality. While comprehensive methodologies for this translation require in-depth exploration beyond the scope of this chapter, this section outlines a phased implementation approach that builds upon the governance foundations established in previous sections.

Phase 1: Diagnostic Assessment (3–4 Weeks)
The implementation process begins with a structured evaluation of organizational readiness across key dimensions identified in Sect. 5.2.5. This assessment examines:

- Existing governance structures and their alignment with the 5P Model
- Priority implementation domains based on identified governance gaps
- Scope definition and integration points within existing institutional frameworks

This initial phase establishes a baseline understanding of the system's current governance maturity, as per the framework presented in Table 5.3, allowing for targeted intervention in subsequent phases.

Phase 2: Value Governance Activation (4–6 Weeks)
Building on the value governance approach detailed in Sect. 5.2.2, this phase focuses on:

- Establishing a multidimensional value framework specific to the implementation context
- Developing governance metrics aligned with strategic priorities

Creating stakeholder engagement strategies for participatory implementationPhase 3: Capability Development (8–12 Weeks)
With governance foundations established, this phase focuses on developing the human infrastructure necessary for sustainable implementation:

- Identifying and developing DBHE competencies appropriate to system maturity
- Implementing core training modules for cross-domain translation
- Establishing mentorship structures for ongoing competency reinforcement

This phase directly addresses the workforce transition challenges identified in Sect. 5.2.1, recognizing that sustainable governance requires not only defined roles but developed capabilities.Phase 4: Operational Integration (12–16 Weeks)

5.3 Beyond Implementation: Building a Global Standard for Digital Behavioral Health...

The fourth phase focuses on embedding governance mechanisms within existing workflows:

- Deploying governance tools aligned with clinical and technical processes
- Establishing feedback mechanisms for continuous improvement
- Developing performance metrics to assess DBHE impact on system outcomes

This integration approach reflects the systems thinking outlined in Sect. 5.2.4, emphasizing that governance must function as operational infrastructure, not separate oversight.Phase 5: Scaling and Sustainability (Ongoing)
The final phase addresses long-term sustainability of the governance transformation:

- Creating knowledge-sharing mechanisms across implementation sites
- Developing certification pathways for DBHEs within existing credentialing structures
- Establishing policy advocacy strategies to secure sustainable funding models

This incremental approach enables health systems to adapt the Global Public Behavioral Health School's core elements to their specific contexts, recognizing that implementation pathways must be responsive to varying levels of digital maturity, regulatory frameworks, and workforce capabilities. Rather than imposing a universal model, the School provides a structured yet flexible framework that can be contextualized while maintaining fidelity to core governance principles.

In line with the ethical frameworks examined in Sect. 5.2.3, this implementation approach emphasizes participatory design at each phase, ensuring governance structures remain responsive to the specific needs and constraints of each implementation context. This adaptive approach acknowledges that governance models must evolve alongside rapidly changing technological capabilities and regulatory frameworks.

As the digital behavioral health ecosystem continues to evolve, implementation will necessarily remain iterative. Initial deployment across diverse health systems will generate comparative data on adaptation strategies, enabling cross-jurisdictional learning while building a global community of practice around digital behavioral health governance. These implementations will particularly focus on identifying minimal viable governance structures that can be deployed even in resource-constrained settings, supporting the value-based approach detailed in Sect. 5.2.2.

The pathway described above represents a systematic approach to institutional transformation—moving from theoretical frameworks to operational governance. Through this structured yet adaptive methodology, the 5P Model and DBHE role transition from academic constructs to practical governance solutions capable of addressing the challenges identified throughout this book.

> While this book offers the strategic architecture for the School, a forthcoming implementation paper will provide a detailed roadmap, including phased deployment, accreditation partnerships, and financing pathways for interested jurisdictions.

5.3.4 Conclusion: From Capability to Commitment

This brief began with a paradox: mental health is both universal and systemically neglected—particularly in digital environments where ethical clarity, operational coherence, and governance capacity are often missing. We proposed that governance—not tools—is the missing infrastructure. Through the 5P Model and the introduction of the Digital Behavioral Health Expert (DBHE), we have outlined a new logic of action that is ethical, scalable, and context responsive.

What began as a response to fragmented accountability and workforce disempowerment has evolved into a governance architecture—participatory by design, distributive by necessity. In this vision, the Global Public Behavioral Health School is not merely an educational institution. It is a strategic coordination mechanism: a way to align localized implementation with shared global standards, enabling culturally adaptive, ethically anchored, and system-aware digital transformation.

This chapter does not offer a final prescription. Instead, it provides a minimum viable roadmap: a set of implementation strategies that can be adapted across systems, geographies, and institutional constraints. Each phase—diagnostic assessment, value activation, capacity development, operational integration, and scaling—has been designed to be both modular and responsive to real-world pressures. These are not abstract steps. They are a call to align intent, capability, and infrastructure.

> This roadmap resonates with Thomas Insel's (2023) five-act trajectory for digital mental health transformation. Insel frames the field's evolution not as a sudden disruption but as a staged process:
> 1. **Act 1: Discovery**—A proliferation of tools and technologies, mostly unregulated, focused on novelty and access rather than clinical integration.
> 2. **Act 2: Definition**—A critical phase in which stakeholders begin to ask hard questions about ethics, equity, standards, and what constitutes "good" digital care.
> 3. **Act 3: Demonstration**—Pilot projects and evaluation frameworks emerge to test effectiveness, contextual relevance, and feasibility.
> 4. **Act 4: Dissemination**—Evidence-based tools are scaled across systems but only if infrastructure, governance, and workforce alignment are in place.
> 5. **Act 5: Deployment**—Full integration of digital behavioral health into standard care, supported by public institutions, ethical oversight, and shared accountability.

(continued)

> Our 5P implementation strategy builds directly on this arc but addresses a critical blind spot: *governance*. While Insel rightly calls for infrastructure, few frameworks define what that infrastructure entails. We propose that ethical deployment (Acts 4–5) is not simply a matter of scaling tools but of building the institutional logic, strategic capacity, and human infrastructure to make digital care safe, equitable, and system aware. The Digital Behavioral Health Expert (DBHE) and the Global Public Behavioral Health School are our proposed vehicles to operationalize this final phase—grounded not only in innovation but in governance by design.

Key Contributions
A reconceptualization of behavioral health governance as infrastructural and anticipatory, rather than reactive or compliance driven

The proposal of the DBHE as a scalable role to orchestrate governance across clinical, technical, and ethical domains

The articulation of the 5P Model as both a policy framework and an operational standard for predictive, preventive, personalized, participatory, and precision-based digital care

The development of a phased implementation roadmap, grounded in systems thinking and institutional design, to guide organizational readiness and workforce transformation

The proposal of a global standard in formation, rooted in codevelopment rather than export and designed to align with diverse governance realities

Limitations and Future Research Directions
This brief is not a finished product—it is a living architecture. Its insights must be tested, adapted, and expanded through practice. Key areas for further inquiry include:

Empirical validation of the DBHE role across diverse health systems, economic models, and sociotechnical environments

Longitudinal assessment of the 5P Model's impact on equity, access, and implementation sustainability

Comparative governance research across jurisdictions to explore interoperability, plural ethics, and policy adaptation

Development of adaptive governance metrics that move beyond clinical throughput or time-based indicators toward multidimensional value measures

An Open Architecture, Not a Closed System
The path forward will not be uniform—but it can be interoperable, participatory, and anchored in public value. We do not offer a universal solution but a modular governance prototype. The DBHE is not a symbolic proposal. It is a trainable, testable, and scalable role, designed for systems that must evolve faster than their current institutional logic allows.

The standards proposed are not fixed—they are open-source, cocreated, and designed to grow through implementation. As such, this brief does not close a conversation. It opens a process: for collaboration, experimentation, and shared learning across sectors and borders.

From Brief to Partnership
This is not just a theoretical framework—it is a structured proposition. If your agency, institution, or system is facing questions around ethical AI integration, digital workforce development, or mental health governance readiness, the next step is not more reading—it is coordinated action. We welcome engagement from partners ready to pilot, adapt, or expand this model.

This is not the conclusion of a model but the commencement of a collaborative journey toward transformative behavioral health governance.

References

Almubarak, L. N., & Alhabeeb, A. A. (2024). The mental health system in the Kingdom of Saudi Arabia. J ISSN, 2766, 2276.
Arefin, S., Zannat, N. T., & Global Health Institute Research Team United States. (2025). Securing AI in global health research: A framework for cross-border data collaboration. *Clinical Medicine And Health Research Journal, 5*(2), 1187–1193. https://doi.org/10.18535/cmhrj.v5i02.457
Auf, H., Svedberg, P., Nygren, J., Nair, M., & Lundgren, L. E. (2025). The use of AI in mental health services to support decision-making: Scoping review. *Journal of Medical Internet Research, 27*, e63548. https://doi.org/10.2196/63548
Bohler, F., Garden, A., Brock, C., & Bohler, L. (2024). Value-based healthcare payment models: A wolf in sheep's clothing for patients and clinicians. *Annals of Medicine, 56*(1). https://doi.org/10.1080/07853890.2024.2382948
Cabitza, F., Campagner, A., & Balsano, C. (2020). Bridging the "last mile" gap between AI implementation and operation: "data awareness" that matters. *Annals of Translational Medicine, 8*(7), 501. https://doi.org/10.21037/atm.2020.03.63
Chakraborty, A., & Karhade, M. (2024). Global AI governance in healthcare: a cross-jurisdictional regulatory analysis. arXiv. https://doi.org/10.48550/arxiv.2406.08695
Damschroder, L. J., Aron, D. C., Keith, R. E., Kirsh, S. R., Alexander, J. A. & Lowery, J. C. (2009). Fostering implementation of health services research findings into practice: A consolidated framework for advancing implementation science. *Implementation Science, 4*(1), 50. https://doi.org/10.1186/1748-5908-4-50
Friedman, C. P., Rubin, J. C., & Sullivan, K. J. (2017). Toward an information infrastructure for global health improvement. *Yearbook of Medical Informatics, 26*(1), 16–23. https://doi.org/10.15265/IY-2017-004

References

Gill, S. P. (2024). Empathy and AI: Cognitive empathy or emotional (affective) empathy? *AI & Society, 39*, 2641–2642. https://doi.org/10.1007/s00146-024-02118-4

Insel, T. (2023). Digital mental health care: Five lessons from Act 1 and a preview of Acts 2–5. *Digital Medicine, 6*(9). https://doi.org/10.1038/s41746-023-00760-8

Iorfino, F., Occhipinti, J. A., Skinner, A., Davenport, T., Rowe, S., Prodan, A., Sturgess, J., & Hickie, I. B. (2021). The impact of technology-enabled care coordination in a complex mental health system: A local system dynamics model. *Journal of Medical Internet Research, 23*(6), e25331. https://doi.org/10.2196/25331

Jeffrey, D. (2016). Empathy, sympathy and compassion in healthcare: Is there a problem? Is there a difference? Does it matter? *Journal of the Royal Society of Medicine, 109*(12), 446–452. https://doi.org/10.1177/0141076816680120

Jaso-Yim, B., Eyllon, M., Sah, P., Pennine, M., Welch, G., Schuler, K., Orth, L., O'Dea, H., Rogers, E., Murillo, L. H., Barnes, J. B., Hoyler, G., Peloquin, G., Jarama, K., Nordberg, S. S., & Youn, S. J. (2024). Evaluation of the impact of a digital care navigator on increasing patient registration with digital mental health interventions in routine care. *Internet Interventions, 38*, 100777. https://doi.org/10.1016/j.invent.2024.100777

Malgaroli, M., Schultebraucks, K., Myrick, K. J., Loch, A. A., Ospina-Pinillos, L., Choudhury, T., Kotov, R., De Choudhury, M., & Torous, J. (2025). Large language models for the mental health community: Framework for translating code to care. *Lancet Digit Health, 7*, e283–e285. https://doi.org/10.1016/S2589-7500(24)00300-1

Marti-Noguera, J. J. (2024). *Ethics in digital mental health: A Comprehensive Guide to Responsible Practice for Professionals in Training*. Ethics Cambridge. International Press. https://ethicspress.com/products/ethics-in-digital-mental-health

Mohr, D. C., Silverman, A. L., Youn, S. J., Areán, P., Bertagnolli, A., Carl, J., Carlton, T., Chaudhary, N., Cooper, D., DeVito, S., et al. (2025). Digital mental health treatment implementation playbook: Successful practices from implementation experiences in American healthcare organizations. *Frontiers in Digital Health, 7*, 1509387. https://doi.org/10.3389/fdgth.2025.1509387

Montemayor, C., Halpern, J., & Fairweather, A. (2022). In principle obstacles for empathic AI: Why we can't replace human empathy in healthcare. *AI & Society, 37*(4), 1353–1359. https://doi.org/10.1007/s00146-021-01230-z

Nair, M., Svedberg, P., Larsson, I., & Nygren, J. M. (2024). A comprehensive overview of barriers and strategies for AI implementation in healthcare: Mixed-method design. *PLoS One, 19*(8), e0305949. https://doi.org/10.1371/journal.pone.0305949

Näher, A. F., Vorisek, C. N., Klopfenstein, S. A. I., Lehne, M., Thun, S., Alsalamah, S., Pujari, S., Heider, D., Ahrens, W., Pigeot, I., Marckmann, G., Jenny, M. A., Renard, B. Y., von Kleist, M., Wieler, L. H., Balzer, F., & Grabenhenrich, L. (2023). Secondary data for global health digitalisation. *The Lancet. Digital health, 5*(2), e93–e101. https://doi.org/10.1016/S2589-7500(22)00195-9

Nilsen, P., Svedberg, P., Neher, M., Nair, M., Larsson, I., Petersson, L., & Nygren, J. (2023). A framework to guide implementation of AI in health care: Protocol for a cocreation research project. *JMIR Res Protoc, 12*, e50216. https://doi.org/10.2196/50216

Nordberg, S. S., Jaso-Yim, B. A., Sah, P., Schuler, K., Eyllon, M., Pennine, M., Hoyler, G. H., Barnes, J. B., Murillo, L. H., O'Dea, H., Orth, L., Rogers, E., Welch, G., Peloquin, G., & Youn, S. J. (2024). Evaluating the implementation and clinical effectiveness of an innovative digital first care model for behavioral health using the RE-AIM framework: Quantitative evaluation. *Journal of Medical Internet Research, 26*, e54528. https://doi.org/10.2196/54528

Robinson, A., Flom, M., Forman-Hoffman, V. L., Histon, T., Levy, M., Darcy, A., Ajayi, T., Mohr, D. C., Wicks, P., Greene, C., & Montgomery, R. M. (2024). Equity in digital mental health interventions in the United States: Where to next? *Journal of Medical Internet Research, 26*, e59939. https://doi.org/10.2196/59939

Strange, M., & Tucker, J. (2024). Global governance and the normalization of artificial intelligence as 'good' for human health. *AI and Society, 39*(6), 2667–2676. https://doi.org/10.1007/s00146-023-01774-2

OECD. (2024). *Futures of global AI governance: Co-creating an approach for transforming economies and societies*. OECD Publishing.

UNESCO. (2021). *Recommendation on the ethics of artificial intelligence*. UNESCO. https://unesdoc.unesco.org/ark:/48223/pf0000381137

World Bank. (2023). *Digital-in-health: Unlocking the value for everyone*. World Bank. http://hdl.handle.net/10986/40212

World Economic Forum. (2021). *Global governance toolkit for digital mental health: Building trust in disruptive technology for mental health* (White Paper). In Collaboration with Deloitte. https://www.weforum.org/whitepapers/global-governance-toolkit-for-digital-mental-health.

World Economic Forum. (2022). *Governance frameworks in digital mental health* (White Paper). https://www.weforum.org/whitepapers/global-governance-toolkit-for-digital-mental-health.

World Health Organization. (2021). *Ethics and governance of artificial intelligence for health: WHO guidance*. WHO. https://apps.who.int/iris/handle/10665/341996

World Health Organization. (2023). *Ethics and governance of artificial intelligence for health: Guidance on large multi-modal models*. WHO. https://www.who.int/publications/i/item/9789240074729

World Health Organization. (2024). *Psychological interventions implementation manual: Integrating evidence-based psychological interventions into existing services*. WHO. https://www.who.int/publications/i/item/9789240087149

World Health Organization. (2025a). *Guidance on mental health policy and strategic action plans: Module 5. Comprehensive directory of policy areas, directives, strategies and actions*. WHO.

World Health Organization. (2025b). *Guidance on mental health policy and strategic action plans: Module 3. Process for developing, implementing, and evaluating mental health policy and strategic action plans*. WHO.

Youn, S. J., Schuler, K., Sah, P., Jaso-Yim, B., Pennine, M., O'Dea, H., Eyllon, M., Barnes, J., Murillo, L., Orth, L., Hoyler, G., & Nordberg, S. (2025). Scaling out a digital-first behavioral health care model to primary care. *Administration and Policy in Mental Health and Mental Health Services Research, 1-21*. https://doi.org/10.1007/s10488-025-01433-2

Glossary

Governance and System-Level Terms

- **Anticipatory Governance**
  A forward-looking governance model integrating foresight, risk management, and participatory engagement to proactively shape emerging technologies and systems.
- **Borderless Digital Ecosystem**
  A digital health infrastructure without geographic or institutional boundaries, requiring governance frameworks that ensure coordinated care, standardized ethics, and interoperable data governance across jurisdictions.
- **Governance Threshold**
  Minimum conditions and mechanisms needed for digital mental health systems to achieve ethical and effective governance beyond mere regulatory compliance.
- **Health Data Space (HDS)**
  Infrastructure designed for ethical data sharing, ensuring governance, compliance, and interoperability across health entities.
- **Hybridity**
  A governance condition in digital behavioral health characterized by simultaneous integration and coordination of overlapping systems—including digital and physical care, public and private platforms, and professional and algorithmic mediation. Hybridity necessitates adaptive governance strategies that reconcile diverse institutional logics, stakeholder perspectives, and operational complexities.
- **Participatory Governance**
  An approach emphasizing active involvement and shared decision-making by stakeholders—including patients, clinicians, policymakers, and technologists—in designing and governing digital behavioral health systems.

- **Participatory Infrastructure**
  Mechanisms and systems facilitating active stakeholder involvement (patients, clinicians, and users) in co-designing, evaluating, and governing digital health solutions.
- **Digital Behavioral Health System (DBHS)**
  An integrated conceptual framework defining digital mental and behavioral health care as interconnected ecosystems rather than isolated apps or fragmented services. The DBHS coordinates technological infrastructures, data governance, clinical practices, ethical standards, and regulatory environments to deliver personalized, preventive, predictive, participatory, and precision-driven mental health interventions at scale.

Clinical, Technical, and Hybrid Concepts

- **Algorithmic Mediation**
  The process by which algorithms actively shape or influence user behavior, clinical decisions, or service delivery in digital mental health. It involves automated decision-making or recommendations requiring ethical oversight to prevent bias, ensure transparency, and maintain clinical quality.
- **Algorithmic Orchestration**
  AI-driven management of workflows, service prioritization, and patient access traditionally executed by human professionals, raising concerns regarding transparency, delegation of clinical authority, and unintended biases.
- **Digital Hybridity**
  The coexistence and mutual influence of analog and digital practices, roles, and infrastructures within mental health systems.
- **Digital Therapeutics (DTx)**
  Evidence-based therapeutic interventions delivered digitally, intended to prevent, manage, or treat mental disorders.
- **Low-Mediation Environments**
  Digital health contexts or platforms with minimal or no professional human oversight, often relying directly on user interaction with automated tools. These environments require embedded transparency and ethical accountability within technological design.
- **Measurement-Based Care (MBC)**
  A clinical approach using frequent, structured data collection (often digitally) to inform and guide mental health treatment decisions.
- **Predictive Psychiatry**
  Application of digital technologies and AI tools to forecast risks or onset of mental health conditions before clinical symptoms become evident.

5P Model and Policy Implementation Terms

- **5P Governance Model**
  A comprehensive governance framework integrating Predictive, Preventive, Personalized, Participatory, and Precision-based principles to ethically guide and manage digital mental health systems.
- **Commodification of Mental Health**
  The transformation of mental healthcare into marketable digital services and products, driven by scalability and cost-efficiency, sometimes at the expense of care quality or ethical standards.
- **Digital Behavioral Health Expert (DBHE)**
  A specialized professional within digital behavioral health governance responsible for integrating clinical expertise, digital technology knowledge, regulatory requirements, and ethical oversight. The DBHE translates the 5P governance model into actionable implementation strategies, ensuring effective, equitable, and ethically sound digital mental health practices.
- **New Primary Care**
  An anticipatory and proactive model of care intervention aligned with WHO people-centered frameworks, emphasizing upstream preventive care, community engagement, and integration of digital transformation within primary health practices.
- **Precision Governance**
  Customizing governance strategies precisely to local needs, ethical considerations, and cultural contexts in digital behavioral health.
- **Structural Hallucination of Economic Implementability**
  A critical term highlighting the flawed belief or illusion that digital solutions alone can sustainably replace traditional mental health workforce models without fundamental systemic and governance reforms.

Ethics, Equity, and Bio-Data Governance

- **Health Equity in Digital Systems**
  Ensuring fair access, usability, and outcomes from digital health solutions across diverse populations, addressing structural, technological, and cultural barriers.
- **Surveillant Prevention**
  A preventive approach relying on continuous monitoring and extensive data collection, shifting responsibility toward individuals rather than system-level accountability, raising ethical and privacy issues.
- **Value Governance**
  An implementation-focused governance logic emphasizing ethical, clinical, and social value creation above traditional productivity metrics. It involves embedding ethical oversight, cultural stewardship, and equitable resource distribution into digital transformation processes.

Implementation and Systemic Learning Concepts

- **Learning Health Systems (LHS)**
  Systems continuously integrating clinical data, user feedback, and research to iteratively enhance care quality, governance responsiveness, and real-time adaptability. LHS support predictive, preventive, personalized, participatory, and precision-based care through continuous learning cycles.
- **Platform Ecosystems**
  Digitally mediated, multi-stakeholder environments enabling shared data governance, collaborative service integration, and participatory management aligned with the principles of the 5P governance model.
- **Sociotechnical Systems**
  Systems deliberately integrating technological solutions and social practices, recognizing their mutual evolution and interdependency.

Emerging Governance and Implementation Concepts

- **Digital Behavioral Infrastructure**
  Platform-based infrastructure replacing traditional analog mental health care, built on predictive analytics, participatory design, and data-driven service integration aligned with the 5P governance framework.
- **Governance Translation**
  The practical competency of converting ethical frameworks, regulatory principles, and theoretical insights into actionable implementation tools, procedures, and governance decisions.
- **Operational Value**
  Measurable and stakeholder-recognized benefits of digital health interventions, extending beyond financial returns to encompass clinical effectiveness, usability, trustworthiness, and broader social legitimacy.
- **Shadow Managers**
  AI-based systems managing service access, scheduling, recommendations, and prioritization in mental health invisibly or with limited transparency, raising significant accountability and ethical oversight concerns.

Index

A
AI in mental health, 88, 95

B
Behavioral health ecosystems, 5, 37, 39, 67, 81, 85, 86, 88, 93, 97, 113, 119
Borderless care, 1–14

C
Cross-sector governance, 83, 86

D
Data-driven systems, 110
Digital behavioral health, 5, 13, 25, 27, 29, 31, 36–43, 81–82, 85–87, 94, 95, 97, 104, 109–111, 116, 120
Digital Behavioral Health Expert (DBHE), 10, 11, 45, 47, 57, 64–75, 81–122
Digital behavioral health governance, 29, 31–45, 61, 64, 71, 104, 107–122
Digital Behavioral Health System (DBHS), 34, 35, 37–43
Digital care transformation, 28
Digital ecosystems, 7, 12–13, 31, 38, 44, 59, 65, 68, 86, 93, 113
Digital governance frameworks, 35–37
Digital transformation, 1–3, 6, 26, 28, 29, 33, 67, 91, 93, 102, 105, 107, 120
Dynamic equilibrium, 1, 14

E
Ethical infrastructures, 64, 117

F
Federated learning (FL), 111–113, 116
5P governance model, 44, 66, 99–101, 116
5P model, 11–14, 21–22, 26, 29, 30, 36, 37, 41–45, 47–75, 81–86, 88, 89, 91, 98–100, 106, 107, 109–111, 118–121

G
Global standards, 7, 72, 74, 107–122

H
Healthcare commodification, 51
Health policy, 13
Health policy transformation, 19–30
Historical evolution, 1–14, 34
Hybrid oversight, 45

K
Knowledge governance, 34, 87, 97

L
Learning health systems, 35–37, 42, 84

M
Mental health economics, 23
Mental health governance, 1–7, 11, 13, 14, 19–30, 47, 50, 51, 75, 83, 86, 102, 103, 122

N
Nation-state paradigm, 1–14

P
Platform-based care, 27
Platform ecosystems, 35–37, 42
Polycentric governance, 38, 40, 100

S
Sociotechnical systems, 35–37, 42, 48, 98

T
Telehealth, 23, 52, 66, 98, 112

V
Value-based care, 52, 75, 82
Value governance, 64, 85, 88–93, 101, 106, 107, 111, 118

W
Workforce transformation, 121

The manufacturer's authorised representative in the EU is Springer Nature Customer Service Centre GmbH, Europaplatz 3, 69115 Heidelberg, Germany. If you have any concerns regarding our products, please contact ProductSafety@springernature.com

Printed and bound by CPI Group (UK) Ltd, Croydon, CR0 4YY
27/03/2026
02080143-0003